MOTIVATIONAL INTERVIEWING
IN THE TREATMENT OF ANXIETY

APPLICATIONS OF MOTIVATIONAL INTERVIEWING

Stephen Rollnick and William R. Miller, *Series Editors*

Since the publication of Miller and Rollnick's classic *Motivational Interviewing*, MI has become hugely popular as a tool for facilitating many different kinds of positive behavior change. This highly practical series demonstrates MI approaches for a range of applied contexts and with a variety of populations. Each accessible volume reviews the empirical evidence base and presents easy-to-implement strategies, illuminating concrete examples, and clear-cut guidance on integrating MI with other interventions.

Motivational Interviewing in the Treatment of Psychological Problems
Hal Arkowitz, Henny A. Westra, William R. Miller, and Stephen Rollnick, Editors

**Motivational Interviewing in Health Care:
Helping Patients Change Behavior**
Stephen Rollnick, William R. Miller, and Christopher C. Butler

Building Motivational Interviewing Skills: A Practitioner Workbook
David B. Rosengren

Motivational Interviewing with Adolescents and Young Adults
Sylvie Naar-King and Mariann Suarez

Motivational Interviewing in Social Work Practice
Melinda Hohman

Motivational Interviewing in the Treatment of Anxiety
Henny A. Westra

Motivational Interviewing: Helping People Change, Third Edition
William R. Miller and Stephen Rollnick

Motivational Interviewing
in the Treatment
of Anxiety

Henny A. Westra

THE GUILFORD PRESS
New York   London

© 2012 The Guilford Press
A Division of Guilford Publications, Inc.
72 Spring Street, New York, NY 10012
www.guilford.com

Printed in the United States of America

This book is printed on acid-free paper.

Last digit is print number: 9 8 7 6 5 4 3 2 1

The author has checked with sources believed to be reliable in her efforts to provide information that is complete and generally in accord with the standards of practice that are accepted
at the time of publication. However, in view of the possibility of human error or changes in
behavioral, mental health, or medical sciences, neither the author, nor the editors and publisher,
nor any other party who has been involved in the preparation or publication of this work war-
rants that the information contained herein is in every respect accurate or complete, and they
are not responsible for any errors or omissions or the results obtained from the use of such
information. Readers are encouraged to confirm the information contained in this book with
other sources.

Library of Congress Cataloging-in-Publication Data

Westra, Henny A.
   Motivational interviewing in the treatment of anxiety / Henny A. Westra. — 1st ed.
      p. cm. — (Applications of motivational interviewing)
   Includes bibliographical references and index.
   ISBN 978-1-4625-0481-7 (hardcover : alk. paper)
   1. Anxiety. 2. Motivational interviewing. 3. Anxiety—Treatment. I. Title.
   BF575.A6.W47 2012
   158.3'9—dc23

2012001799

To Bill and Steve for their pioneering efforts

To my dear colleagues at York (and Mike)
who regularly inspire me

To Joanne, Clarence, Meisje, and Jenny
for their unconditional love

To my parents for their support

And to Carl Rogers,
the grandfather of motivational interviewing

About the Author

Henny A. Westra, PhD, is Associate Professor of Psychology at York University in Toronto, Ontario, Canada. She has extensive clinical and research experience and has worked as a front-line clinician, clinical director, professor, and trainer. She is a member of the Motivational Interviewing Network of Trainers (MINT). Dr. Westra's research on motivation and interpersonal process in psychotherapy has been funded by the National Institute of Mental Health and the Canadian Institute of Health Research. She has presented and published widely on the treatment of anxiety and depression.

Series Editors' Note

The field of motivational interviewing (MI) is moving fast. Rising publication rates across diverse areas reflect the attentiveness not only of researchers, but of clinicians too. This book combines both sensibilities, in a new area of application.

The orientation of this text will serve the field well. MI emerged from humanistic and behavioral psychotherapy, and in the face of so many efforts to adapt it for use by practitioners outside of these fields, this book returns you to its roots. Henny Westra pays very careful attention to the therapeutic relationship and to what happens in a conversation about change. These are the twin threads that run through any use of MI, and they are woven together with considerable skill in this text. The book shines with clinical experience.

The clients Westra writes about are mostly help-seeking, and they often present with interrelated problems, whatever label is attached to them. Westra breaks new ground in demonstrating how to discuss complex problems without oversimplification, and with a clear sense of direction: resolution that promotes growth and freedom from tension, distress, and disability.

This book arrives at a time of transition in our own writing on MI, shortly before the third edition of our text appears (Miller & Rollnick, in press), yet the evidence of synergy with our work is striking. Westra's journey into what she calls the action stage is well matched by our own thinking on what we call the planning process. Put simply, talk about planning involves skillful attention to the language of change, as does helping someone resolve ambivalence and move toward decision making.

"MI makes good clinical sense," one of Westra's closing comments in this book, is a phrase that captures much of what precedes it. This book lays down a challenge to clinicians to be thoughtful and skillful, and to researchers to study process in addition to client outcomes. We congratulate and thank her for making such considerable experience available to others.

STEPHEN ROLLNICK
WILLIAM R. MILLER

Preface

SCOPE AND OVERVIEW OF THE BOOK

Since its inception, motivational interviewing (MI) has diffused rapidly. It was originally developed within the area of problem drinking as an alternative to the confrontational style of interaction that often characterized addictions counseling at the time. Since then, MI has become an established, empirically supported treatment for substance abuse, has been extended to health behaviors, and is more recently being applied to the treatment of other major mental health problems such as anxiety disorders, eating disorders, depression, problem gambling, and corrections.

This book describes the integration of MI with other therapies for the treatment of anxiety and co-occurring problems such as depression. I consider what treatment for these problems would look like if it were informed by MI. A major aspect of MI is a specific attitude held by the therapist—a particular way of thinking about the client, the process of change, and the therapist's role in it. This "MI spirit" draws heavily on the client-centered therapy and principles outlined by Carl Rogers, and MI principles and methods derive from this foundational attitude, with specific MI techniques representing opportunities to communicate this attitude.

My objective in this book is not to identify what is lacking in other major approaches to treating anxiety but rather to suggest (from my own particular vantage point) how treatment might be enhanced if it were informed by knowledge of MI. I suspect that many good therapists will recognize themselves and what they do (perhaps intuitively) in these pages.

This effort is an attempt to show how MI can make explicit some of what may have previously been implicit or unspecified.

WHO SHOULD READ THIS BOOK?

This book is intended for any helping professional involved in providing a formal course of treatment for those with anxiety and related problems. This target group includes practitioners working within many other major approaches to therapy, and this volume may be especially useful for those working with more directive or action-oriented approaches for promoting behavior change. It focuses on anxiety and the problems that go along with it, most notably depression, since these are highly prevalent problems in clinical practice and therefore provide an essential context for illustrating how MI can inform other treatments. Whether anxiety constitutes the primary reason for treatment or accompanies other problems, this book is intended to provide guidance on how infusing treatment with MI can advance client engagement and treatment response. Practitioners of various approaches will improve their skills at recognizing and effectively managing ambivalence and motivational impasses that often threaten the client's efforts to change.

Many of the clinical illustrations in the book will be most familiar to individuals practicing cognitive-behavioral therapy (CBT). This is because my background is in CBT, and my primary orientation in clinical practice is the integration of MI with specific CBT methods and concepts. However, since the MI-informed elements of therapy presented in this book are not intended to be specific to any particular orientation, interventions derived from other approaches can be substituted for the specific methods used for illustration.

A BEGINNING EFFORT

This book is one of a number of attempts to describe how MI can inform the process of treatment more broadly (with the COMBINE trial in the area of substance abuse being another [COMBINE Study Research Group, 2003]; see also Arkowitz & Burke, 2008, on integrating MI into the treatment of depression). Other approaches exist that outline how a client-centered perspective can serve as an essential platform from which a variety of more directive interventions and approaches can be practiced (emotion-focused therapy: Greenberg, 2002; Greenberg, Rice, & Elliott, 1993; client as self-healer: Bohart & Tallman, 1999). Accordingly, this book represents an initial effort to integrate MI specifically with other more action-oriented methods. I suppose I am in a unique position to make an initial attempt at such an integration since I have a foot planted in several different worlds, including CBT, MI, and client-centered principles,[1] and thus can appreciate the strengths and limits of each of these major models.

I hope this book encourages you to seek training in MI (or, if you already know MI, enables you to extend the application of it to common problems like anxiety); enhances your practice, whatever your approach; and stimulates thinking and dialogue about how client engagement with existing approaches can be improved.

---

[1] With deep gratitude to my client-centered colleagues at York University, from whom I have learned a great deal, especially Lynne Angus, John Eastwood, Leslie Greenberg, David Rennie, and Shake Toukmanian.

Contents

PART IV. EXTENDING MOTIVATIONAL INTERVIEWING
INTO THE ACTION PHASE

PART V. PUTTING IT ALL TOGETHER

Integrating Motivational Interviewing into the Treatment of Anxiety and Related Problems

1

෨

Where and Why
Motivational Interviewing Fits

Constant or overwhelming feelings of worry, fear, and dread can create great suffering and misery for those who are repeatedly hijacked by anxiety. When severe enough, it is common for anxiety (and the accompanying search for safety) to eclipse critical priorities such as educational or career advancement, forming satisfying relationships, and leisure pursuits, or more generally feeling joy and contentment. It is also not uncommon to see people limping along in their jobs, relationships, or activities but feeling chronically distressed, unsatisfied, or even depressed. Such feelings often prompt people to consider treatment.

While one might assume relief from these highly noxious feeling states would be incentive enough to work toward overcoming them, people are surprisingly conflicted about being less anxious or depressed and about taking action to bring about these ends. Change is difficult and fraught with ambivalence, including conflicting and often opposing motives and feelings. Individuals with anxiety commonly wrestle with such ambivalence. While they may be aware that anxiety is causing problems and have a desire to be free from it, familiar patterns have a seductive quality, despite the many problems they may create. Moreover, it is difficult and demanding to face one's fears, a necessary step in overcoming anxiety, and this is typically not done without significant reluctance and reservations.

Although motivational interviewing (MI) was originally developed as a method to help people work through conflicted feelings about drinking, it is also highly relevant and adaptable to the treatment of anxiety and related problems. Having the tools to help clients process their mixed feelings about change, in an atmosphere of acceptance and understanding, enables a ther-

3

apist to help clients more confidently and effectively move toward change. And MI is now striking a chord with helpers seeking to facilitate change in many different domains and with many different populations.

My own attraction to MI arose from my experience in working primarily within a cognitive-behavioral orientation to treat those suffering with anxiety and depression. I saw the enormous value of cognitive-behavioral therapy (CBT) for many clients, but for others this approach seemed to fall flat. Realizing that CBT strategies worked very well if a client used them, I began to advocate more vigorously for their adoption by my less engaged clients—with predictably poor results. Rather than increasing their willingness to change, my attempts at advocacy for CBT seemed to alienate my clients further. These interactions would often end in argument, frustration (on both sides), and therapeutic impasses. Moreover, the clients I struggled with would continue to occupy my thoughts in a way that my motivated clients did not. My exposure to MI offered me a complementary skill set that I did not possess at that time. Most critically for me, MI offered a humane and more satisfying way of viewing behavior and working in harmony with my clients, rather than wrestling with them. And this approach, although initially intended for the treatment of substance abuse, seemed to be highly relevant and valuable in navigating the ambivalence about change that I routinely saw in working with those suffering from anxiety and depression.

In recent years, issues of treatment nonadherence and noncompliance have taken center stage. Helpers working in many areas, from medication adherence to lifestyle change to alleviating the suffering of those

> *MI offers a humane way of viewing behavior and working in harmony with clients, rather than wrestling with them.*

with anxiety and related problems, are increasingly observing the pernicious problem of lack of client engagement with change, even when help is available and offered. In some ways it seems counterintuitive that clients, even in the presence of great suffering and a clear desire for change, would resist change. Why would people not do what is—even to them—clearly in their best interests? In such a situation it is natural to assume, as I previously did, that clients lack knowledge and direction. Perhaps they don't know how to change.

Let me recount some recent experiences that I had with helpers in my own life when writing this book, in order to position MI in the context of common, intuitive approaches to accomplishing behavior change. When I went to see my family physician for my annual checkup, he quite matter of factly told me that I should use less salt—use it either while cooking or sprinkle it on top of food while eating, but not both. What he didn't seem to appreciate or inquire about however, was my deep love of salt and all things salty. And he seemed to assume that correcting my information gap (although I was already aware of the potential health dangers of excessive salt) would be enough to elicit my compliance. After all, this was for the good of my health.

Then I joined a gym where the fitness assessor seemed slightly more aware of issues of noncompliance. She explained that many people join the gym but then stop coming after a time—a situation she admitted she was at a loss to understand. She stressed that she could only give me the information and point me in the right direction but that it was up to me to decide whether to comply. Although she was explicitly acknowledging my freedom to choose and the words sounded right, something was missing. I was left feeling that she was either attempting to coerce me or didn't really care if I complied. Clearly helpers of all stripes, while recognizing the need to improve engagement with treatment, are struggling to figure out how to accomplish this and are often ineffective, despite their well-intentioned efforts.

In a sense, it is striking that we have developed so many effective strategies and approaches to help clients with anxiety accomplish change and yet we have neglected a fundamental truth that everyone from lay people to clients to trained professionals readily acknowledges: that change is impossible unless one wants to change. And once sufficient interest and motivation for change are present, change seems far less difficult and daunting and tends to proceed far more smoothly. As articulated by Sheldon, Williams, and Joiner (2003), clinicians who are technically proficient and knowledgeable about methods of facilitating change or action will often find themselves impotent if they are unable to build motivation and help clients work through their conflicting, powerful, and often contradictory feelings about change.

In this book, I suggest that efforts to get people to change, such as those of my family physician and my fitness appraiser, are destined to fail if they are devoid of relationship and context—of interest in the person, their reactions, life circumstances, preferences, beliefs, and values. Through situating attempts to explore and build motivation for change in the context of the person and a secure therapeutic relationship, MI offers a uniquely engaging way forward to facilitating client active involvement with treatment and change, one that is complementary to more action-oriented approaches that are prevalent in the treatment of anxiety and related problems.

In this chapter, I briefly describe the major anxiety disorders and their current treatment. I then consider why it makes sense to integrate MI into the treatment of anxiety and

> *We have developed effective strategies to help clients change anxiety, but change is impossible unless one wants to change.*

commonly co-occurring problems such as depression, and provide an overview of this proposed integration.

OVERVIEW OF ANXIETY DISORDERS AND THEIR TREATMENT

There are several major types of anxiety disorders (see Barlow, 2002, for a more complete elaboration). In descending order of prevalence, they include:

- Specific phobia or fear of circumscribed objects or situations (e.g., heights, injections, flying). Even though specific phobias are the most prevalent type of anxiety, they are less likely to present to treatment than the other types of anxiety, which are typically more complicated, distressing, and impairing.
- Social phobia (fear of embarrassment or humiliation in social or public situations).
- Posttraumatic stress disorder (PTSD; persistent reexperiencing of a traumatic event, distress associated with exposure to reminders of the event, and emotional detachment)
- Generalized anxiety disorder (GAD; excessive, uncontrollable worry in a number of areas such as health, work performance, the well-being of others, finances, etc.).
- Agoraphobia (fear of being unable to escape or of being alone in the event of a panic attack).
- Panic disorder (recurrent unexpected panic attacks—sudden escalation of multiple somatic fear symptoms such as heart racing shortness of breath) which is often associated with the development of agoraphobia.
- Obsessive–compulsive disorder (OCD; recurrent and intrusive thoughts, images, or impulses such as fears of contamination or thoughts of harm toward others and/or repetitive actions aimed at reducing anxiety or neutralizing obsessive thoughts).

All anxiety disorders involve bodily arousal, threat-related thoughts and beliefs, and avoidance, each influencing the others to maintain the experience of anxiety (Dozois & Westra, 2004). While the focus of the threat differs among the various types of anxiety, anxious arousal is triggered by external cues (e.g., needles in injection phobia, social situations in social anxiety, reminders of the traumatic event in PTSD) or internal cues (e.g., heart racing or dizziness, obsessive unwanted thoughts, worry itself) that signal the presence of threat. These situations are given catastrophic appraisals (e.g., heart racing may be interpreted as indicative of an impending heart attack or death in panic disorder, social interaction may represent the possibility of shame or embarrassment in social anxiety), and the client experiences a sense of having limited personal control over the feared events, hypervigilance or chronic anticipation of encountering feared situations, and attention narrowing to concentrate on the focus of threat.

All anxiety disorders involve attempts to take protective actions to reduce threat and reestablish safety. Most typically these involve attempts to escape or avoid feared stimuli, with the particular pattern of avoidance being consistent with the specific situations that are feared. While outright avoidance of feared situations is common, many attempts at avoidance are more subtle. For instance, a person may remain in a frightening situation but initiate behaviors (e.g., using alcohol, carrying safe objects) or thought processes (e.g., distraction, mental rehearsal) to dampen the anxiety and worry (Dozois & Westra, 2004). Unfortunately, these attempts at avoidance serve to perpetuate the very anxiety from which one seeks relief. They reinforce the perceived danger of the threat and perpetuate a lack of self-efficacy or control in managing the threat. Avoidance also serves as negative reinforcement (temporary alleviation of anxiety). In essence, by avoiding, the person fails to learn some basic truths about potential dangers: that negative predicted events do not always occur, and, even if they do, that they are manageable and not as disastrous as the anxiety predicted.

Prevalence of Anxiety and Associated Problems

Anxiety disorders are the most common of all mental disorders, with high 1-year and lifetime prevalence rates of 17% and 25%, respectively (Kessler et al., 1994). They are associated with much distress, suffering, and related problems, and, if left untreated, anxiety disorders tend to persist and recur. Studies of quality of life among individuals with anxiety disorders reveal a picture of marked impairment in many areas, including educational and career development, employment, and relationships (Mendlowicz & Stein, 2000). In fact, the reduced quality of life reported in individuals with anxiety disorders is comparable to, and in some instances worse than, major medical illnesses (e.g., Rubin et al., 2000).

An individual with an anxiety disorder often has other associated mental health problems, most commonly depression, other anxiety disorders, and substance abuse (Barlow, 2002). Most striking is the relationship between anxiety and depression. About 50% of those who have an anxiety disorder are also depressed (Brown, Campbell, Lehman, Grisham, & Mancill, 2001), and this rate climbs to 76% when considering lifetime diagnoses (Brown & Barlow, 2009). Anxiety is also more likely to precede depression than the reverse (Brown et al., 2001; Cole, Peeke, Martin, Truglio, & Seroczynski, 1998). The extensive overlap between anxiety and depression has raised questions as to whether they are distinct syndromes (Barlow, 2002). Accordingly, treatment protocols that consider the commonalities among the anxiety disorders (e.g., Norton & Hope, 2005) and between anxiety and depression (e.g., Ellard, Fairholme, Boisseau, Farchione, & Barlow, 2010) have emerged recently. In short, anxiety disorders are common, often associated with marked impairment, distress, and reduced quality of life, and without treatment they tend to persist.

Treatment of Anxiety

Effective treatments for anxiety disorders have been developed, most notably CBT (Barlow, 2002; Norton & Price, 2007). Large effects in reducing symptoms have been consistently reported across numerous well-controlled studies. Various treatment guidelines now recommend CBT as the first-line approach to treating anxiety disorders (e.g., National Institute of Clinical Excellence, 2004; Swinson, 2006).

Although CBT treatments typically consist of multiple types of interventions (e.g., self-monitoring, cognitive restructuring, relaxation training), most emphasize exposure to feared situations/stimuli as a critical and necessary component of treatment. By facing, confronting, and remaining in threatening situations, a client can extinguish fear, experience new learning, and develop more adaptive coping skills, reducing the need to avoid feared situations in the future. Reductions in the threat occur as new evidence is accumulated that differs from catastrophic predictions. Hence, heavy emphasis is placed on helping the person to approach feared situations. In general, exposure to unwanted, aversive, and avoided experiences is a common goal in approaches to treating anxiety.

WHY APPLY MOTIVATIONAL INTERVIEWING TO ANXIETY?

Ambivalence about Change

Ambivalence about change is extremely common, even among those who have decided to enter treatment. In fact, up to two-thirds of individuals entering treatment for mental health problems can be classified as being in either the precontemplation (not yet actively considering change) or the contemplation (considering change but conflicted) stage of change. That is, they are significantly uncertain or undecided about change and therefore are unlikely to use action-oriented strategies (O'Hare, 1996). While people desire change, they simultaneously fear it. Existing patterns and ways of being have a seductive and compelling quality and frequently threaten and sabotage efforts to change. As Mahoney (2003) has noted, many of the processes that we see as pathological are actually efforts at self-protection and cohesion and therefore can be highly resistant to change. Research with those suffering from anxiety suggests that many individuals enter treatment reluctantly and with significant reservations about engaging with therapy (e.g., Dozois, Westra, Collins, Fung, & Garry, 2004; Simpson, Zuckoff, Page, Franklin, & Foa, 2008). For example, among those with OCD considering treatment, Purdon, Rowa, and Antony (2004) found that 94% of their sample articulated at least one treatment-related fear. The most common fears included concerns about intensifying anxiety and fears of failure in treatment, rendering the individual more hopeless. Other concerns included fear of success (resulting in increased expectations from others) as well as fears of disclosure and therapist judgment. Such fears of treatment have been identified as a major cause of the failure to seek help for mental health problems (e.g., Kushner & Sher, 1989). That is, individuals contemplating seeking help must balance their desire for symptom relief against potential concerns about, and the costs of, seeking help.

Individuals who worry excessively often see worry as a problem while simultaneously holding positive beliefs about worry (e.g., "Worry is motivating," "Worrying protects me and prepares me for negative events") and are therefore ambivalent about relinquishing it (e.g., Borkovec, 1994; Westra & Arkowitz, 2010). Even something as noxious as rumination, which is common in depression, can be perceived as a positive attempt to find answers or understand past mistakes and failures (Papageorgiou & Wells, 2001). Moreover, self-blame, self-criticism, and withdrawal are often familiar response styles learned as a way to cope with environmental and interpersonal stress, and are adaptive and "safe" behaviors when in conflict with powerful others, such as early attachment figures (Gilbert & Irons, 2005). At times, such defensive strategies will bring temporary relief. Similarly, there is a high degree of ambivalence among individuals who contemplate suicide; they want to die, but they also want to live with less pain (Jobes & Mann, 1999). And the ratio of the strength of the wish to live to the wish to die is a critical determinant of future suicide-related behavior (Kovacs & Beck, 1977).

Resistance in Therapy

Much of what is thought of as resistance or noncompliance in psychotherapy may be a reflection of this ambivalence about change (Engle & Arkowitz, 2006). This may explain why many clients remain in treatment but either fail to comply or comply only minimally with recommended treatment procedures. For example, homework assignments are frequently recommended across various types of psychotherapy, and in some forms of treatment (such as CBT) they are regarded as essential. However, homework noncompliance is a common clinical reality. In surveys of practicing CBT therapists, deviations from the assigned task are commonplace, with only a minority of clients identified as totally compliant (Kazantzis, Lampropoulos, & Deane, 2005). And homework noncompliance has been described as the rule rather than the exception in CBT (e.g., Helbig & Fehm, 2004). Moreover, resistance to therapist direction has been identified as a strong predictor of both subsequent engagement with the tasks of treatment (Jungbluth & Shirk, 2009) and outcome (Aviram & Westra, 2011; Beutler, Harwood, Michelson, Song, & Holman, 2011).

Treatments that direct clients to take action toward change require a relatively high level of client motivation. Thus, limited engagement with treatment among those who are ambivalent about change may be at least partially responsible for limiting response rates to these treatments. For example, despite the well-established efficacy of CBT in the treatment of anxiety and depression, a substantial number of patients do not engage or respond adequately (e.g., Westen & Morrison, 2001). In a survey of expert CBT practitioners, the most frequently cited reasons for insufficient treatment response were, by a wide margin, "lack of engagement in behavioral experiments" and "noncompliance" (Sanderson & Bruce, 2007). Strong convergent evidence has emerged for the importance of resistance to change and treatment as an important process marker indicating the use of supportive rather than directive strategies (e.g., Beutler et al., 2011), with the addition of MI substantially reducing resistance in CBT for anxiety (e.g., Aviram & Westra, 2011). And active involvement in and receptivity to the treatment process is consistently related to better outcomes (e.g., Orlinsky, Grawe, & Parks, 1994).

The Evidence for Motivational Interviewing in the Treatment of Anxiety

Even though MI is a well-supported treatment in the substance abuse domain (e.g., Hettema, Steele, & Miller, 2005) and it seems to make sense to integrate it into the treatment of anxiety and related problems such as depression, research has only recently begun to test the value of adding MI to existing treatments for these conditions (Westra, Aviram, & Doell, 2011). Consistent with the early stage of this work, this research includes uncontrolled case studies and controlled pilot studies. Case study data supporting adding MI and motivational enhancement strategies including MI have been reported for a range of anxiety disorders, including OCD (Simpson & Zuckoff, 2011), GAD (Westra & Arkowitz, 2010), social anxiety disorder (Buckner, Roth Ledley, Heimberg, & Schmidt, 2008), panic disorder (Arkowitz & Westra, 2004), health anxiety (McKay & Bouman, 2008), and mixed anxiety and depression (Westra, 2004). In studies that have compared MI to psychoeducational or no-treatment controls, MI is demonstrating promise in:

- Increasing treatment seeking among those with social anxiety who are not yet seeking care (Buckner, 2009).
- Increasing problem recognition and treatment attendance for PTSD (Murphy, 2008).
- Increasing receptivity to recommended treatments such as exposure and response prevention for OCD (McCabe, Rowa, Antony, Young, & Swinson, 2008; Tolin & Maltby, 2008).
- Improving response to CBT for anxiety more broadly (Westra & Dozois, 2006) and GAD in particular (Westra, Arkowitz, & Dozois, 2009)

In a larger controlled trial of adding MI (or no MI) as a pretreatment to CBT for GAD, MI was found to substantially improve worry reduction among those with the most severe worry at the outset of treatment (Westra et al., 2009). In this study, those of high worry severity who received MI as compared to those who did not, showed substantially lower levels of resistance (i.e., higher receptivity to change) in CBT, and this accounted for their higher levels of worry reduction in treatment (Aviram & Westra, 2011). While promising, these studies have a number of important limitations, and future research, using rigorous controlled designs, is needed to determine the value of adding and/or integrating MI with other treatments for anxiety and depression.

Research on the use of MI to manage depression is still in the very early stages. A number of supportive uncontrolled case studies using MI for depression (Arkowitz & Westra, 2004; Brody, 2009) and suicidal ideation (Britton, Patrick, Wenzel, & Williams, 2011; Britton, Williams, & Connor, 2008; Zerler, 2009) have been reported. Swartz and colleagues (2006) developed and examined the impact of an engagement interview, which drew heavily on MI principles, with mothers of psychiatrically ill children (who suffer from very high rates of mental health problems, especially depression, yet rarely seek treatment). In one study, among the 13 individuals who received the interview, 85% went on to complete the subsequent treatment (interpersonal therapy for depression) and showed significant improvement (Swartz et al., 2006). Similar findings with another difficult-to-engage population—pregnant, depressed, economically disadvantaged women—have also been reported. In this study, 68% completed a full course of treatment as compared to only 7% of the usual care group (Grote et al., 2009).

Even a brief dose of MI (10–15 minutes) resulted in higher levels of engagement with an Internet-based treatment designed to prevent depression among at-risk adolescents, compared to brief advice from their primary care physician (Van Voorhees et al., 2009). Similarly, Simon, Ludman, Tutty, Operskalski, and Von Korff (2004) used structured MI exercises to enhance engagement of depressed primary care patients in telephone CBT, finding that this group showed lower depression scores as compared to those receiving treatment as usual. Finally, Britton and colleagues (2011) have recently adapted MI to address suicidal ideation (MI-SI). MI-SI is a single-session treatment designed to access and enhance clients' motivation to live and engage in life-enhancing activities. This treatment was reported to be well tolerated, but the intervention has yet to be tested for its efficacy in improving treatment retention and outcomes in controlled studies.

TWO WAYS TO USE MOTIVATIONAL INTERVIEWING

In this book, I suggest there are two major ways to use MI in the treatment of anxiety and related problems: (1) using MI to build motivation among those who are significantly ambivalent about change and (2) using MI as a foundational framework for guiding those who are ready to take action toward change.

Using Motivational Interviewing to Build Motivation

One way of integrating MI in treatment involves using it in the face of high levels of client ambivalence about or resistance to change. And this represents the way that MI has typically been thought about and used: to build resolve or momentum to change in the presence of ambivalence about and resistance to change. For example, it may be clear from the initial interview or early in treatment that specific attention needs to be paid to building motivation for change. A client may express skepticism or ambivalence about change, have previously failed in attempts to change, or have low expectations for being able to change. Alternatively, motivational impasses may arise (or recur) when the client is taking action to change. For example, a client may oppose therapist suggestions or show low levels of engagement with in-session or between-session tasks. At these times, shifting out of an action-oriented approach and into MI temporarily may be useful until client motivation and engagement with the tasks of change are established (or reestablished).

Thus, MI can be used as a pretreatment and/or integrated into more action-oriented treatments when motivational impasses occur. These are the most common ways that MI has been thought about and utilized, and they seem to be particularly indicated when clients are "stuck" and resist active efforts to change. Indeed, in a recent study of client accounts of their experiences of MI for worry, the largest dimension that emerged was reports of increased resolve, momentum, and determination to change (Marcus, Westra, & Angus, 2011). Furthermore, evidence suggests that MI is synergistic with other therapies; that is, the effects of MI are stronger (Burke, Arkowitz, & Menchola, 2003) and more enduring (Hettema et al., 2005) when it is used in an adjunctive capacity.

One major objective of this book, then, is to extend the application of MI to the treatment of anxiety and the problems with which it commonly co-occurs. To this end, I describe and illustrate the application of MI to building motivation and enhancing resolve for change among those suffering with various anxiety disorders, as detailed by the original developers of MI, William Miller and Stephen Rollnick (2002). Strategies for building motivation can be used whenever resistance and ambivalence emerge over the course of treatment. Accordingly, in Part II of this book, Assessing Readiness for Change, various ways of recognizing ambivalence and resistance are outlined. Such skills are necessary in order to identify when the strategies for building resolve and increasing motivation are indicated and, more generally, to build sensitivity to hearing resistance to change and to promote flexibility in responding to it. Part III, Understanding Ambivalence and Building Resolve, outlines the application of MI to building motivation and enhancing commitment to change among those with anxiety and related problems. Specifically, the MI skills of understanding ambivalence (Chapter 5), reframing resistance to change (Chapter 6), evoking and elaborating change talk (Chapter 7), and developing discrepancy (Chapter 8) are discussed in the context of work with anxiety and related problems.

Using Motivational Interviewing Beyond Building Motivation

Although MI is typically thought of as a method to build motivation, it does not have to end there. That is, a clinician does not have to pick up MI to enhance motivation for change and then put it down again once the client seems ready to change. Upon learning MI, you begin to see other possibilities for fitting it into your broader practice, such as:

- Being more evocative generally (e.g., stopping before answering a client's question in order to have the client answer it first).
- Explicitly recognizing clients' autonomy to choose, even when they are committed to change (e.g., often saying "Only you can know what is best").

- Becoming more sensitive to hearing how clients talk about change (developing a kind of radar for resistance whenever it arises, including during the action phase).
- Starting to think about your role differently (i.e., as more of a guide rather than an expert teacher) even when the client is taking action.
- Appreciating the subtleties and complexities of the gentle, powerful art of reflective listening and how it can be used to advance planning for and processing change (realizing for example, that how you reflect things can lead someone to further elaborate or back away from a previous statement or position).
- Generally finding yourself becoming increasingly sensitive to how engaged the client is with the process of treatment, on a moment-to-moment basis, over the entire course of therapy.

All of these things are consistent with MI, and learning MI can change you. It can make you more sensitive, not only to issues of motivation and resistance to change but also to client engagement and disengagement with the process of treatment. It can also make you more sensitive to how you present things and how you come across in therapy and, more broadly, to the significance of the underlying interpersonal and communicative process that occurs between client and therapist.

Perhaps because of this heightened sensitivity, you find yourself working in harmony with your clients more often or even most of the time (even when you're not "doing MI") and experience the process of therapy to be a real partnership where each person contributes valuable expertise. If you are less familiar with client-centered therapy (on which MI is based) and were trained in a more directive model of therapy, learning MI can heighten your awareness of the significance, difficulty, power, and complexity of skills like empathic listening, providing unconditional positive regard, rolling with resistance, and, more broadly, developing a safe and collaborative therapeutic relationship. You begin to wonder (and sometimes struggle) about how such skills can be integrated into your practice more broadly, even when motivation is not an issue.

> Learning MI can change you as a clinician.

Thus, in addition to enhancing motivation, there may be other possibilities for integrating MI into treatment. In particular, MI has much to tell us about the underlying interpersonal process of therapy or *how* treatment can be conducted. MI rests on the foundations of client-centered counseling (Rogers, 1951, 1957, 1965), described in MI language as "MI spirit," which refers to a particular attitude or way of being with clients. Accordingly, this spirit is considered more critical than any particular method within MI (see Chapter 2). Indeed, when you talk to MI practitioners, you realize that what is shared in common more than anything else is a way of thinking—a particular way of looking at people, change, and one's role in this process. The impact of this attitude can be most readily observed in the interpersonal process between client and therapist. It informs or translates into a particular manner in which the therapist interacts with clients (e.g., evoking client expertise and strengths, recognizing and safeguarding client autonomy, avoiding power struggles, and the like).

In this sense then, *MI can serve as a foundational framework into which other treatments can be integrated.* This extension of MI to supporting action toward change naturally emerges from the underlying spirit or attitude of MI. This spirit constitutes a platform or framework that informs how more action-oriented therapies might be conducted. Thus, combining the client-centered spirit of MI (ways of being) with the technical merits of other treatment approaches (ways of doing) may constitute a meaningful and powerful point of integration. Moreover, a wide variety of specific intervention methods to promote behavior change can be integrated into, or conducted from, an MI stance. This may be particularly the case since MI was not originally intended as a standalone therapy and makes no claims about which strategies are superior for achieving behavior change (Miller & Rollnick, 2009).

Significant advances have been made in developing effective interventions for helping those suffering with anxiety and depression to achieve relief from these debilitating conditions. Action-oriented treatments such as CBT (e.g., Barlow, 2002), acceptance and commitment therapy (Hayes, Strosahl, & Wilson, 2012), mindfulness awareness (Segal, Williams, & Teasdale, 2001), and behavioral activation (Martell, Addis, & Jacobson, 2001), among others, have repeatedly demonstrated their efficacy as treatments for anxiety and co-occurring problems of depression. While the importance of collaboration, empathy, and the therapeutic alliance have clearly been acknowledged in these approaches, less attention has been paid to proficiency in the relational aspects of therapy as compared to technical proficiency with specific interventions.

In other words, many action-oriented treatment protocols are typically better at specifying *what* to do rather than *how* to do it. That is, describing the underlying interpersonal process and therapist attitudes conducive to effective intervention are less well specified. Arguably, the relational context in which change strategies are presented and implemented is an important determinant of client receptivity to them. And specific interventions or change methods can never be disembedded from their relational and communicative context. Importantly, extending the MI relational stance (and the methods that emerge from it) into the action phase of therapy can avoid some of the pernicious problems of resistance and noncompliance that more directive approaches can often create.

Variability in relational skills may be an important area that accounts for therapist variability in outcomes despite similar levels of technical competence (e.g., Huppert et al., 2001). It may be likely that those therapists who are more proficient in generating positive outcomes by using action-oriented treatments are more relationally adept (e.g., sensitive to resistance and alliance ruptures, flexible, empathic, attuned to fluctuating client needs and engagement, warm). For example, more-effective CBT therapists are characterized by clients as more client-centered (evocative, collaborative), while less-effective therapists are described as more compliance-oriented and as prioritizing their own expertise (Kertes, Westra, & Aviram, 2010). And CBT therapists who go on to generate clients high in expectations for a positive outcome show vastly better skill at maintaining a friendly, collaborative atmosphere in the presence of client opposition or disagreement than those therapists whose clients went on to be pessimistic about treatment outcome (Ahmed, Westra, & Constantino, 2010).

In other words, what may differentiate more- from less-effective action-oriented therapists is the underlying attitude of the therapist or the interpersonal spirit in which treatment takes place. This conclusion is echoed by colleagues who have often observed, "Good therapists [practicing my particular approach] are sensitive to relationship and client engagement issues and flexible in response to fluctuating client motivation." Arguably, these underlying process variables need to be explicitly specified and operationalized, especially if they are skills capable of differentiating success and failure with a particular treatment. And MI may provide a vehicle for specifying, at least in part, an effective process for conducting therapy.

Thus, with respect to the second way to use MI, Part IV of this book, Extending Motivational Interviewing into the Action Phase, presents some ways in which MI can inform treatment even when ambivalence about change is not (or is less) present. Specifically, I discuss and illustrate methods for evoking, building, and elaborating client expertise in envisioning, planning for, and processing efforts to change (Chapter 9). I also discuss means of bringing in therapist expertise while protecting and reinforcing client autonomy (Chapter 10). In addition, I suggest a major role for empathy and listening reflectively in the action stage to accomplish common and important goals in the treatment of anxiety and related problems, including self-confrontation, exposure to avoided experience, and promoting self-acceptance (Chapter 11). Finally, I outline the MI strategies for rolling with resistance and illustrate their use with clients in the action stage of therapy to process the natural fluctuations that occur in client resolve to take action (Chapter 12).

SUMMARY AND CONCLUSION

In short, ambivalence about treatment and change is common in clinical practice, including among those seeking relief from anxiety and depression. Most people come to therapy in great pain, and often they are confused and conflicted about the origins of this pain and what they want to change. This ambivalence may give rise to resistance, noncompliance, or limited and reluctant engagement with taking action to change. Noticing this often profound ambivalence, and working with it while abstaining from imposing one's own agenda, preferences, values, and desires, is a key part of MI.

Research on MI for anxiety and related problems is just beginning, but existing evidence is consistent in supporting the potential of MI to enhance engagement with and response to other treatments including CBT (Westra et al., 2011). It is particularly promising that MI is demonstrating efficacy with populations (treatment refusers, those reluctant to seek care) and subsets of populations (e.g., high severity) that are typically treatment-non-responsive and difficult to engage. Moreover, the key clinical skills of MI such as empathy, cultivating a positive therapy relationship, and flexibility in responding to fluctuating client needs are important contributors to client benefit from therapy generally, and these skills seem to be especially indicated when navigating ambivalence and resistance.

As such, integrating methods to address ambivalence, reduce resistance, enhance intrinsic motivation, and prepare people for change complements more action- or change-oriented approaches to the treatment of anxiety. I have argued that this can be done in two ways: (1) through using MI (as originally conceived) to enhance motivation among those who need this and (2) through extending the underlying spirit and methods of MI into the action phase to help clients conceptualize, plan for, implement and process the changes they wish to make. Doing so may not only improve the effectiveness of major approaches to the treatment of anxiety and related problems such as depression but also facilitate training in the process factors and therapist attitudes that most influence client engagement with therapy.

2

∞

The Spirit
of Motivational Interviewing

In his 1951 book *Client-Centered Therapy*, Carl Rogers begins by discussing the importance of the attitude underlying client-centered practice:

> The counselor who is effective in client-centered therapy holds a coherent and developing set of attitudes deeply embedded in his personal organization, a system of attitudes which is implemented by techniques and methods consistent with it. How do we look upon others? Do we respect [the individual's] capacity and right to self-direction, or do we basically believe that his life would be best guided by us? Are we willing for the individual to select and choose his own values, or are our actions guided by the conviction (usually unspoken) that he would be happiest if he permitted us to select for him his values and standards and goals? (Rogers, 1951, pp. 19–20)

In MI, this underlying client-centered attitude is referred to as the "MI spirit," and it permeates, informs, and underlies every clinical encounter. At its core, MI rests on a particular view of human nature, the client, the change process, and the therapist's role in facilitating that change. This means that MI cannot be distilled into a set of questions or techniques one can memorize and regurgitate. Any therapist behavior, no matter how much it may resemble MI, is not considered MI unless it is congruent with this underlying attitude.

Use of specific techniques in MI without the underlying spirit is like "words without music" and is not MI (Rollnick & Miller, 1995). This may be one of the reasons why MI without a manual tends to be more effective than structured MI with a manual (Hettema et al., 2005). That is, MI is fundamentally a "way of being" with clients, which in turn infuses and guides every therapist action and communication, both verbal and nonverbal.

Stated differently, in MI, therapist actions can be thought of as the means through which a particular view of the individual and the process of change is communicated. Every therapist action communicates something to the client. And techniques can never be divorced from the relational context in which they are expressed, including the underlying attitudes of the individual implementing the techniques. In MI, it is not so much the techniques themselves that are important but rather what they convey.

Every therapist action communicates.

MI IS NOT THE SUM OF ITS PARTS

MI cannot be equated with any particular method, and it is more than the sum of its constituent parts. Any technique is merely an expression or instantiation of the underlying spirit and objectives of MI. For example, even decisional balance, a technique with which MI is often (incorrectly) equated, is not an *exercise* that one completes and is not even mandatory. Rather, it is merely a convenient and potentially useful heuristic for advancing the therapist's (and therefore the client's) understanding and exploration of ambivalence about change.

Consider the following clinical illustration that reflects the common temptation to distil MI into a set of techniques. A trainee I was supervising began therapy with a client who presented with excessive worry and depression. Given that the client had been in treatment without success on two previous occasions and presented as skeptical (e.g., questioning various aspects of the treatment process), we agreed that MI to enhance motivation was indicated. The trainee thus dutifully set out to do MI (memorizing questions and directions from various readings assigned to him). He articulated that the session failed to take off or get traction and there was trouble establishing a focus. When we watched the tape together, it became clear that the trainee was more preoccupied with doing MI (and doing it well) than "simply" listening and being present with the client.

After checking my impression against the trainee's experience in the session, I encouraged him to begin with reflective listening and then watch for the presence of ambivalence (ambivalence as a marker), should it arise. Almost immediately, the client indicated that she felt stuck since she was hanging on to a previously terminated relationship with her ex-boyfriend and had recently attended one of his therapy sessions to explore the possibility of reuniting with him. She noted enormous internal conflict between the logical part of her brain, which said that she should let go of him and "move on," and her feelings, which were compelling her to not abandon the possibility of a relationship with him. Thus, in this instance, the therapist worked far more productively by focusing less on technique and more on cultivating a therapeutic attitude that included openness to being directed by the client.

There is an onus on the counselor practicing MI to know, cultivate, and nurture MI spirit—and to monitor deviations from it. In terms of learning MI, this means that one would do better to grasp the client-centered attitude underlying MI than to focus on learning specific techniques. Indeed, while there are many variations on technique, the underlying spirit is more enduring and therefore a more reliable compass from which to navigate the counseling process.[1]

Miller and Rollnick (2002) have elaborated how the MI spirit and the methods that flow from it can be used to resolve ambivalence as well as enhance motivation and commitment to change. In this book, I consider how MI can be used to accomplish these goals when working with anxiety and related problems (in Parts II and III). In addition, I argue that the MI spirit and the methods grounded in it do not have to be restricted to building motivation but rather can also be extended to accomplish major tasks of treatment with these populations. Such tasks include increased self-awareness, self-confrontation, exposure to avoided experiences, and carrying out experiments in behavior change (see Part IV). Thus, in exploring how MI can inform the treatment of anxiety and related problems, we must begin with an understanding of this underlying spirit.

MOTIVATIONAL INTERVIEWING SPIRIT

Client as Expert

Before outlining the client-centered spirit underlying MI, it may be useful to understand how the assumptions underlying MI are different from the assumptions of the model guiding many therapy approaches in practice today, the medical model.[2] As summarized by Bohart and Tallman (1999),

---

[1] This is consistent with the emphasis in client-centered and related experiential therapies on therapist presence and the cultivation of therapeutic attitudes in the therapist (Geller & Greenberg, 2002; Rogers, 1980).

[2] Valuable and more extensive elaborations contrasting the medical model with client-centered or contextually-sensitive approaches are available from Bohart and Tallman (1999) and Wampold (2001).

In the medical model, the therapist is analogous to the physician. He or she is the expert on the nature of the client's problems and on how to remediate those problems. He or she forms a diagnosis of the client and then prescribes treatment. Treatment consists of applying interventions appropriate to that diagnosis. These interventions cause change in the client, thereby alleviating the symptom. (p. 5)

Accordingly, the primary responsibilities of the patient in this model are to recount information (so that the doctor can accurately diagnose and then formulate a treatment plan) and to actively comply with the recommended treatment. The relationship between doctor and patient in the traditional medical model is important mainly in increasing patient compliance with treatment; it operates strategically as a means to an end. Most therapy approaches that are oriented toward helping clients take action to change would accord a greater role for collaboration in therapy than this description implies. Nonetheless a power imbalance often exists, with the therapist regarded as possessing the expertise to promote behavior change and the client as the recipient and beneficiary of this expertise. In contrast, in MI the client is not viewed as deficient or lacking expertise that the therapist then supplies. Rather, clients are seen as already possessing all they need to resolve ambivalence and accomplish change. The MI therapist trusts this and seeks to identify and mobilize these intrinsic resources in order to stimulate behavior change. Motivation is seen as coming from within and can never be supplied from without. Recognizing this, the MI therapist consistently communicates, "I don't have what you need, but you do. And I will help you to find it." Thus, the MI therapist resists the temptation to supply expertise to correct client deficiencies and resists assuming he or she knows what clients need to do to resolve problems and live more satisfying lives. The therapist actively avoids holding such agendas for clients and instead seeks to identify and work with the client's priorities, ideas, and preferences.

This approach is often surprising for clients, who readily defer to others owing to a lack of confidence in their own abilities to make decisions, take effective action, or pursue satisfying directions in their lives. The therapist's belief in and approach to the client as fully capable is a crucial antidote to the typical lack of self-regard and self-efficacy often seen in clients who struggle with anxiety and depression. The therapist's belief in the client's ability to navigate the way forward fosters greater client self-belief, self-trust, and self-efficacy. That is, the therapist's consistent acts of trust in the client's inherent wisdom and innate abilities translate into greater client self-trust.

Let me provide a clinical example of the sometimes powerful nature of this "client-as-expert" attitude to be therapeutic in and of itself. I recall working with a client who had a strong conviction that any form of weakness, vulnerability, or frailty was unacceptable—to herself and others. She greatly feared that any expression of weakness or reliance on others would cause others to lose respect for her. Much of her life was focused on the effort to be strong, invulnerable, protective of others, and reliable. And yet she constantly deferred to others (including frequent efforts to flatter me and solicit my expertise), reflecting an inner sense of failure to trust her own intuitions and resources. I recall a particularly poignant moment in which the client remarked that "I have *so* much respect for you." I sincerely responded, "And you know what, Rose, I have enormous respect for you as well." The client became tearful and shook her head, remarking, "But I'm sitting in *this* chair"—reflecting the very active core belief that "people can't respect me if I am vulnerable, have problems or weaknesses." I replied that we could flip a coin to decide who would sit in which chair; but, given that she was paying me, I probably should continue to occupy the therapist's chair. In this instance, I refused to see the client as "weak" or "fragile" despite her having problems and also refused her attempt to elevate my status above her own. This created a powerful discrepancy with her existing expectations ("others will look down on me if I show weakness") and served as a catalyst for a new and more adaptive view of herself in relation to others. Thus, the egalitarian attitude of MI—the inherent belief in and respect for clients' capabilities, despite their own lack of trust in themselves—can be healing in and of itself.

> The therapist's belief in the client is an important antidote to how the client views him- or herself.

Challenges to Assuming the Client-as-Expert Stance

For those (like myself) more familiar with action-oriented approaches, adopting a client-as-expert attitude can represent a formidable and challenging perspective shift, since the therapist's role is to provide what the client is presumed to be lacking (e.g., coping skills, information). For example, one therapist learning CBT whom I was training had a strong "teaching" style with little room for client involvement. I suggested to him that he consider being more evocative by asking clients more often what they thought. The therapist replied: "I can't do that. What if they give me the wrong answer?"

Assuming a client-as-expert stance can be especially challenging when clients expect or pressure you to be the expert and actively solicit and defer to your expertise in providing advice and solutions. In the famous tape of Carl Rogers working with Gloria (Rogers & Shostrom, 2000), when Gloria repeatedly asks Rogers to tell her what to do, Rogers acknowledges Gloria's deep desire to have an answer and notes that, although he can't supply an answer, he will surely help her to find her own answers. Such an approach communicates the therapist's conviction that the client inherently possesses the solutions and that, with persistence, patience, and focused exploration of the problem, the answers the client is seeking will emerge. Miller and Rollnick (2002) refer to this as "resisting the righting reflex." That is, when clients present problems, MI therapists resist the temptation to fix them.

Indeed, clients and therapists alike can harbor underlying assumptions of the counseling process that prize the therapist's perspective and interventions in bringing about change. Recently, in my undergraduate counseling class, I asked students to complete the Helpful Responses Questionnaire (Miller et al., 1991), which asks them to respond with what they would say next to a number of different client problem presentations. All 26 would-be counselors provided specific "helpful" advice (sometimes adamantly) on how to go about resolving the various problems presented, and only one student made any attempt to understand or express empathy. Client expressions of suffering can give rise to a strong impulse among helpers to take away that suffering, and these often lead to explicit therapist recommendations on how to do so.

In interpersonal terms (e.g., Kiesler, 1996), a client's suffering can come across as an expression of submission (to the therapist's expertise and superior knowledge), which automatically and forcefully pulls for a complementary response of therapist dominance. The client's underlying message (sometimes explicitly expressed) is: "I'm incapable. I can't figure it out. I need someone else to do that." The client's suffering can also communicate either an inability to tolerate the process of self-exploration or the experience of emotional pain (i.e., "I can't stand what I'm feeling—you need to take it away"). And if such messages are met with the "righting reflex," it unfortunately can have the effect of reinforcing clients' beliefs in their lack of capabilities or capacities for emotional tolerance and self-righting resources. Although this approach derives from compassion and a wish to alleviate suffering, following this instinct can block important opportunities for clients to discover their own solutions and to realize that they can be trusted to do so.

Here, it is important to remember that the process of searching, self-examination, and discovery can be more important than having "answers." Honoring that difficult process can communicate important therapeutic messages in itself (e.g., tolerating distress and uncertainty, the value of compassion and patience). I recall working with a client who was trying to sort through a decision about whether to end his recent marriage. He repeatedly expressed frustration at himself for having created the situation (marrying his wife despite strong doubts about the wisdom of doing so) and for his general paralysis in being able to take action to resolve it. In one session in particular, I recall working hard to cultivate an attitude of patience, a recognition that the situation was complex and that there are no easy answers to complex problems. And I explicitly congratulated him for considering all the various aspects and implications, reframing his not knowing as wise avoidance of a quick decision and as reflecting his caring and conscientiousness. I asked the client at the end of that session how he felt. He replied, "I still don't know what to do, but somehow that feels more okay right now."

There can be a fear in learning and practicing MI among therapists used to more action-oriented approaches that they will lose an important source of expertise. This is likely especially frightening for therapists (like myself) who have developed and honed their skills in precisely identifying and diagnosing clients' problems (for the purpose of applying specific treatments to resolve those problems). I recall a pivotal experience when I was just beginning to learn MI. I asked a client what she would recommend to someone just like herself if she were this person's therapist. Her responses could have filled a best-selling self-help book. I recall distinctly being demoralized by this and questioning why I got a degree in clinical psychology if people already knew how to change. I ultimately came to realize that for many individuals the issue is not "how" to change but rather how to manage the internal obstacles and ambivalence that get in the way of acting on that inherent knowledge.

What Does One Do Instead of Supplying Expertise?

So, if one resists the righting reflex, doesn't that leave a vacuum? What do we do to help the client move toward behavior change? Where does our expertise reside? So far, we have seen what we should *not do*; so, what then *do* we do? Indeed, client-centered approaches are often described as laissez-faire, passive, and lacking direction. Therapists can fear that if they resist supplying particular expertise on problem resolution, they will be doing nothing. As we will see in the chapters that follow, MI is far from nondirective, empathic reflection and related skills within MI are far from passive, and there are particular ways of contributing your unique knowledge or expertise that preserve the client's autonomy rather than undermining it.

In MI, the emphasis is on creating the conditions that allow clients to solve their own problems—creating the atmosphere or climate that allows clients to productively work toward resolving ambivalence and mobilizing resolve and resources for change. In this sense, when working from a client-centered framework and attitude, *one is not so much an expert on the content of the problems or their resolution (that is the client's domain), but rather one is an expert on the process.* Interestingly, in Rogers's reply to Gloria's request for advice, he not only says what he cannot do (namely, give her a solution) but also what he can do—journey together with her to help her find the answers she so eagerly desires (Rogers & Shostrom, 2000). Accordingly, in MI it is up to the client to talk him- or herself into change, resolve ambivalence, and explore one's own beliefs, ideas, desires, values, and solutions; the job of the therapist is to create the conditions in which this self-discovery becomes possible.[3]

So, what are these favorable conditions? Like client-centered therapy, MI stresses the essential importance of the development of a safe collaborative space in which the client can sort out his or her confusing, conflicting, and often contradictory views of change. Here the relationship is viewed as a supportive context and workspace in which the client, together with the support and resources the therapist brings, can use his or her own active intelligence to engage in generative thinking processes. In this sense, MI converges with the client-centered tradition of prioritizing the therapeutic relationship as an essential vehicle in which greater self-awareness can be developed and new meanings generated. Rogers's emphasis on the importance of the therapeutic relationship has since been supported by decades of research on the importance of relatedness, including research on the therapeutic alliance (Constantino, Castonguay, & Schut, 2002; Horvath & Symonds, 1991), attachment (Cassidy & Shaver, 2008), and the necessity of caring, affection, and interpersonal safety for facilitating exploration and new learning (Gilbert, 1993, 2010).

More than just technical expertise, therapists bring themselves—their humanity—to the encounter. They bring their curiosity, compassion, understanding, and validation. They bring faith in the process and in the capacity of everyone to be free from suffering and live a meaningful, satisfying life that is congruent with their values. They protect the clients' rights to self-determination and freedom from coercion and offer themselves as confident companions and guides in their clients' journeys of self-discovery and, ultimately, behavior change.

Stated differently, MI is primarily discovery-oriented (rather than "teaching"-oriented). It seeks to create the conditions under which preexisting client creativity and capability can be uncovered and unleashed in the service of change. As such, therapy often has an emergent quality as clients explore and find sources of motivation, identify key needs and values, and discover new alternative perspectives and possibilities. Through their belief in clients, their curiosity, and their evocativeness, MI therapists seek

---

[3] Similar views stressing the capacity and resources of the client, with therapists mobilizing, evoking, and working with these resources, have been articulated by others (e.g., Bohart & Tallman, 1999; Duncan, Hubble, & Miller, 1997; Orlinsky et al., 1994).

to stimulate such discoveries and to elaborate them to create new energy and resolve for achieving change.

MI is primarily discovery-oriented.

Working in Harmony with the Client

Given the significance of creating and maintaining the therapeutic relationship and the atmosphere of discovery, MI therapists seek to work in harmony with clients at all times. They avoid coercion, argumentation, confrontation, or even persuasion. These styles of interacting emerge from a therapist-as-expert frame and they run the risk of engendering client resistance. And even small amounts of resistance have a strong capacity to negatively affect outcomes (Aviram & Westra, 2011; Jungbluth & Shirk, 2009; Westra, 2011).

The MI therapist continually monitors interactions for evidence of disharmony, noncollaboration, and working at cross-purposes and seeks to respond to such signals of resistance to reestablish harmony. MI therapists are sensitive to how they present their inputs to the process (whether questions, reflections, suggestions, interventions, or education) in order to maximize clients' receptivity to them. MI therapists aim to avoid pressuring clients, interrupting their processes, or threatening their autonomy. Concomitantly, they also monitor clients' receptivity and seek to continually modify and refine their efforts to maintain clients' engagement.

At moments of disharmony, MI therapists avoid pejorative perceptions of clients as unmotivated, obstructive, or difficult. They seek to reframe clients' resistance by working and siding with it, understanding it, and finding the wisdom in it. In fact, sustained client noncompliance or resistance to therapist direction is not considered a client problem in MI but rather a therapist skill error. Resistance reflects valuable self-protective instincts that are to be honored and worked with in the service of exploring and implementing change.

MOTIVATIONAL INTERVIEWING
PRINCIPLES AND METHODS

Putting Motivational Interviewing Spirit into Practice

Thus far, we have discussed the spirit or attitude underlying MI. What does this look like in practice? What are the therapist behaviors that flow from this spirit? As an evolution of the client-centered therapy elaborated by Carl Rogers (1951, 1956, 1965, 1975), MI emphasizes empathic understanding of the client's internal frame of reference. Miller and Rollnick (2002) define MI spirit as consisting of three major dimensions: collaboration, evocation, and preservation of client autonomy. In addition to expression of empathy, these constitute the major dimensions on which adherence to MI is judged (Moyers, Martin, Manuel, Hendrickson, & Miller, 2005).

Collaboration refers to working together in harmony with the client. While all therapeutic approaches strive to create a collaborative environment, in MI these efforts flow from the particular view of the client and the change process that constitutes the spirit of MI. There is no power imbalance in MI. Rather, the therapist works to cultivate an egalitarian relationship where each member contributes valuable expertise. Accordingly, MI therapists avoid the use of persuasion and confronting clients with their point of view.

Since motivation for change and client resources in bringing about change are presumed to already exist, the MI therapist seeks to draw out these innate resources. The emphasis is not on installing what is missing but rather on evoking what is existing; not on imparting therapist expertise but on uncovering client expertise; not on providing prepackaged answers to problems but on discovering solutions together. The therapist contributes an active interest in supporting and helping clients articulate their own ideas regarding change. In MI, it is the client and not the therapist who articulates the reasons for change and resolves ambivalence about change. This is often a bottom-up or emergent process that requires patience— watching, waiting, listening for, seeking, and creating opportunities to elicit client ideas about change and the process of change. Thus, MI therapists actively avoid imposing their own views of reasons for change. They do not educate or give opinions without being invited. And they hold their own ideas lightly and are prepared to relinquish them—recognizing the client's authority as the final and sole arbiter of all decisions regarding change.

Relatedly, particular and explicit emphasis is placed on recognizing and *protecting client self-determination and autonomy.* The MI therapist believes the client is the only authority on decisions regarding change, and these can never be appropriated by another—no matter how well intentioned. MI therapists accept that clients may choose not to change, may avoid or delay change, or may proceed with change in an unconventional manner (or in a manner that differs from the preferences of the therapist). The MI therapist recognizes and conveys an understanding that the critical variables for change are within the client and can never be imposed by others. That is, motivation arises from personal goals and values and not from external sources (including the therapist).

Thus, MI is not coercive or "strategic," that is, *not a clever way of getting the client to do what you want him or her to do.* In fact, such controlling and coercive attitudes are antithetical to the spirit of MI. The MI therapist recognizes, and relates to the client, that choices always reside with him or her. Pressuring and persuading clients to act in accordance with the therapist's aspirations and needs introduces contingencies in the relationship (i.e., conditional positive regard—"I will like and accept you if you do this or think that . . . but not if you don't"). Even if one "gains compliance" (i.e., the client submits or relents), this "choice" is now confounded by the client's need to maintain harmony in the therapeutic relationship and may not reflect consistency with his or her own intrinsic direction. The clinician practicing MI actively becomes aware of and lets go of any personal motivations or aspirations for clients in order to be open to exploring the client's goals, motives, and aspirations.

Another way in which the client's autonomy and authority is communicated is through the use of tentativeness (e.g., "I'm not sure about this . . .," "This may or may not fit for you . . .," "If I hear you right, you are saying . . .") and encouraging the client to check therapist inputs (e.g., through reflections, feedback) against his or her own experience. Essentially the attitude is one of "See what you think of this and check it against your own experience, ideas, and preferences, because what *you* think—not what *I* think—is the most important thing here." The implicit message is that the therapist can never possess the truth about the client, can only ever guess about the client's experience, and can offer useful input only if the client is open to hearing it. The client is the ultimate arbiter of decisions regarding whether and how to change. Accordingly, MI is not something one does "to" a client but rather "with" him or her.

The Four Principles of Motivational Interviewing

Further specifications on successfully enacting MI spirit are reflected in the four principles of MI. These represent major aspirations of the MI therapist in promoting resolution of ambivalence about, and ultimately commitment to, change (and, as we will see, these can be extended to accomplish goals in the action phase of therapy). These aspirations include expressing empathy, developing discrepancies, rolling with resistance, and supporting self-efficacy.

Expressing empathy involves striving to understand and experience the world (particularly emotions and meanings) from the client's perspective, without judgement or criticism, and continually reflecting this emergent and evolving understanding back to the client. This quiet eliciting process can appear slow and passive, and often it looks deceptively simple, particularly if one is used to taking a more directive approach. However, empathic listening is a highly active, complex, and multilayered process that is critically important in helping clients understand and work through ambivalence about change. Moreover, as a vehicle for promoting self-awareness and encouraging self-confrontation, empathic listening can play a central role in accomplishing vital tasks of treatment in the action phase of therapy. MI also involves *developing discrepancies* between the client's intrinsic values, objectives, and desires, on the one hand, and their current behavior, on the other. Arguably, the need to act in accordance with one's values is a major incentive for change and can provide the momentum to resist the forces supporting the status quo. Since individuals strive for consistency in their beliefs and behavior, heightening awareness of how the current behavior thwarts realization of personal goals produces discomfort, which the client naturally seeks to resolve. For example, a client who values his relationship with his children will find it unsettling to realize how his overprotectiveness alienates his children. Helping clients develop greater awareness of their values can also serve as positive incentives or valued directions to strive toward. This generates not only inconsistency and discomfort to be resolved but also a positive motivational force through envisioning a desired future (Wagner & Ingersoll, 2008).

Greater awareness of the client's values and goals can be a powerful ally, not only in helping the client to resist the forces of the status quo but also as the client begins experimenting with new ways of being that are more consistent with his or her values. For example, in this latter phase, the therapist can help the client experiment with new value-consistent behaviors (e.g., being assertive) and to process the outcome of these experiments in terms of their feel and "fit" with respect to core intrinsic values (e.g., to express one's own needs and desires) rather than externally imposed or introjected values (e.g., to meet the needs of others, or to be consistent with what one "should" do).

In MI, therapists *roll with resistance* by seeing it as a reflection of valuable information to be understood rather than an obstacle to be overcome. They side or work with it, rather than against it. In MI, resistance to change is defined as the product of both the client's ambivalence about change and the way the therapist responds to this ambivalence (Moyers & Rollnick, 2002). A substantive body of research supports resistance as an important process marker in therapy requiring the use of supportive rather than directive approaches. When building resolve to change, rolling with resistance can involve developing awareness and understanding of the often powerful forces for the status quo (resisting change) rather than working to defeat these forces. In the action phase of therapy, it can involve sensitive attunement and supportive responding to moments of client opposition to change or disharmony in the therapy relationship.

Finally, MI therapists seek to *enhance and support client self-efficacy*. MI is a strength-based approach that helps clients identify their own existing intrinsic wisdom, creativity, and resources for resolving problems. People often have the necessary knowledge and resources to accomplish change once they have overcome the inertia of ambivalence. By eliciting and supporting the activation of the client's own ideas, preferences, and resources, the MI therapist seeks to strengthen the client's agency (i.e., the belief that he or she can effectively accomplish the changes he or she desires to make). Such skills can be used not only for eliciting motivation for change but also for evoking clients' resources, ideas, and preferences for developing and refining plans and steps toward change.

Increasing Change Talk

Informed by recent research on the role of clients' language in MI, particular attention is paid to client speech and therapist behavior in shaping it (Miller & Rose, 2009). The proficient use of MI should ultimately increase client's in-session "change talk" (talk in the direction of change) and decrease their "sustain talk" (talk in favor of not changing). Experimental studies have demonstrated that MI substantially lowers resistance to change (Aviram & Westra, 2011; Miller et al., 1993) and increases change talk (Miller et al., 1993) relative to control conditions. Linguistic analysis of MI session tapes (Amrhein, Miller, Yahne, Palmer, & Fulcher, 2003) have demonstrated a particular progression of client speech in good outcome sessions in substance abuse populations. In particular, client articulations of desire, ability, reasons, and need for change have been found to precede client commitment, with the pattern of commitment statements uniquely predictive of subsequent behavior change. In particular, increasing strength of commitment over the course of a session was found to predict abstinence.

Thus, in building resolve to change, when sufficient motivation is present, the therapist shifts to strengthening commitment to change and converting motivation into commitment to specific change goals and plans. Moreover, as we will see, sensitivity to client verbalizations reflecting movement toward or away from change (i.e., how clients talk about change) and using these as markers to inform therapist responses (in an effort to nurture or increase change talk and movement toward change) continue to be very important skills in the action phase of therapy.

SUMMARY

The client-centered spirit on which MI rests involves a view of the client as having innate recuperative capabilities. A major task of therapy from an MI perspective is to create the relational climate in which these abilities can be called forth and harnessed in the service of behavior change. The specific principles and methods of MI can be considered means of enacting this underlying spirit and communicating this particular view of the individual.

In short, in MI, clients are regarded as the best experts on themselves. They have the freedom to make their own choices and an intrinsic knowledge of what is best for them. The therapist operates as an evocative consultant or guide (Rollnick, Miller, & Butler, 2008) in the client's journey. The aim is to respect the self-propelled growth process in the individual, understanding that when the conditions are right the person will move in positive life-affirming directions. In essence, through a belief in clients' innate but undiscovered capacity for self-healing and self-determination, MI therapists seek to help clients *recognize themselves as an authority*. They promote and support clients' active use of that authority to make choices, informed by a heightened awareness of their own best interests, values, and valued directions.

MI, then, consists of relational (ways of being) and technical (ways of doing) components. MI therapists are intentionally and consciously directive in facilitating deeper client understanding of the competing forces surrounding change; in creating greater awareness of client inherent values, desires, and preferred directions regarding change; in reflecting and heightening discrepancies between these valued directions and current behaviors; and more generally in listening for, nurturing, and guiding clients to elaborate and build their intrinsic motivations for change. Through being sensitively attuned to the client and recognizing and respecting the client's authority, MI seeks to tip the balance in favor of promoting and supporting change. This attitude (MI spirit) and the specific methods flowing from it serve as the fuel for helping clients work through their ambivalence about and resistance to change. And, as we will see, this attitude (and the methods that emerge from it) can be extended to supporting and facilitating clients' persistence in taking action to accomplish the changes they desire.

PART II

ℭ

Assessing Readiness for Change

3

Observing Resistance

You might have noticed that a particular intervention can be "solid gold" with one client but fall totally flat with the next client. Or a statement ("Therapy can be quite effective for your problem") offered when a client has a high level of motivation will likely be welcomed and foster hope but may be precisely the wrong thing to say when a client has doubts about treatment (and will likely yield a "Yes, but . . . "). Thus, timing and client readiness for change are crucial contextual determinants of receptivity to, and consequently the efficacy of, interventions.

Prochaska (1999) identifies two major errors in the process of facilitating change. The first is encouraging action when the client needs to contemplate (i.e., is not yet ready to take action), and the second is encouraging contemplation when the client needs to act (i.e., is ready to act). Similarly, Miller and Rollnick (2002) stress the importance of shifting to supporting action toward change when this is indicated by the client's level of readiness. Thus, motivation and, more broadly, observations of client engagement in the process of therapy are key elements of the therapy context that require continual monitoring as a basis for selecting the most effective clinical approach. And acquiring sensitivity to hearing these changing conditions on a moment-to-moment basis is important to using both more supportive and more directive styles effectively. This is particularly important since motivation can wax and wane over the course of therapy, and responding flexibly to these shifts in change readiness is an important clinical skill.

In this chapter and the next one, I discuss two major methods of assessing client readiness to change, observing readiness (this chapter) and asking about readiness (next chapter). These methods are offered as guides for determining how to respond in a way that matches your client's readiness level. After briefly discussing different clinical styles in the absence and presence of resistance, I elaborate on developing the capacity to listen

> *Continual monitoring of client engagement is essential in selecting the most effective approach.*

for and hear the client's expressions of readiness or lack thereof as they occur on a moment-to-moment basis in therapy sessions. Such observations can include attentiveness to client opposition to therapist inputs and direction (resistance in process) as well as client statements regarding change (resistance in language). Finally, more broadly, therapists can observe other signals of client readiness, including experimenting with change, reduced discussion of the problem, and so on. The next chapter provides some questions that can be asked in an interview and reviews a number of self-report scales that can provide useful clinical information in determining whether to begin with building motivation (Part III) or proceed to helping the client develop an action plan and supporting him or her in enacting this plan (Part IV).

THE IMPORTANCE OF MINIMIZING RESISTANCE BY SHIFTING CLINICAL STYLES

Research has demonstrated that resistance to the therapist can be toxic to maintaining a strong sense of collaboration in therapy and to therapy outcomes. For example, sessions rated by clients as being low in therapy alliance have been observed to contain significantly higher levels of resistance to the therapist as compared to those rated by clients as high in therapy alliance (Watson & McMullen, 2005). Higher levels of resistance, even as early in the therapy as the first session, tend to strongly predict subsequent engagement with the tasks of treatment and ultimately overall benefits from therapy for anxiety (Aviram & Westra, 2011) and depression (Jungbluth & Shirk, 2009). And even though early resistance was quite rare in these studies relative to cooperation, it was capable of strongly predicting subsequent engagement (homework completion and involvement in therapy sessions) and outcomes. This set of findings suggests that moments of opposition may represent key moments in the therapy process that need to be attended to immediately and navigated successfully to reduce their negative impact. This interpretation is consistent with reviews of the literature on resistance, which conclude that there is strong evidence that the effectiveness of therapy is associated with the relative absence of resistance (Beutler et al., 2011; Beutler, Moleiro, & Talebi, 2002a, 2002b) and the quality of the client's engagement with treatment is among the most critical contributors to treatment outcomes (Orlinsky et al., 1994). Thus, minimizing resistance and maintaining a high level of engagement in therapy are important process goals of therapy.

The good news is that therapists can exert a powerful impact on client levels of resistance. That is, resistance is not static but rather the product of a client's ambivalence and how a therapist responds to this ambivalence (Moyers & Rollnick, 2002). Therapist directiveness has been found to reliably increase client resistance, while supportive and self-directed approaches reduce it (e.g., Aviram & Westra, 2011; Beutler et al., 2002b; Miller et al., 1993). For example, Patterson and Forgatch (1985) had therapists alternate within a session between teach and confront, on the one hand, and facilitate and support, on the other. The former increased resistance, while the latter evoked greater cooperation. Directiveness may be helpful in certain contexts, such as when the client is cooperative, but detrimental in the presence of resistance and ambivalence, when supporting the therapeutic alliance becomes especially significant (Beutler, Harwood, et al., 2011; Beutler, Moleiro, et al., 2002a, 2002b; Ilgen, McKellar, Moos, & Finney, 2006).

As such, the ability to hear client resistance and disengagement and to shift out of being more directive in the presence of doubts about treatment and change is very important. For example, Burns and Auerbach (1996) note that continuing to use cognitive therapy in the context of client anger or noncompliance can convey the message that the patient's perceptions are irrational or ridiculous. Rather, they argue, "When patients are stuck or angry or expressing strong negative affect, therapists need to set their cognitive and behavioral techniques temporarily on the shelf and respond in an empathic manner" (p. 150). Arkowitz and Westra (2004) note that, if change-oriented strategies are used in the context of strong ambivalence about change, "The therapist risks being perceived by the client as an advocate for change (i.e. hearing only one side of their ambivalence), similar to the stance often taken by significant others (e.g. family members, doctors). In this sense the client and therapist are 'acting out' the client's ambivalence." Finally, in a study of therapist behaviors contributing to ruptures and their repair in the therapy relationship in CBT, Aspland, Llewelyn, Hardy, Barkham, and Stiles (2008) concluded that, on noticing an alliance rupture, CBT therapists should become more empathic and responsive, switch their focus to issues more salient to clients, and encourage clients to express their concerns rather than continuing with technical interventions.

Moreover, there is now also evidence that responding with support rather than direction in the presence of resistance may generate higher levels of optimism about change (a factor common to all therapy approaches that is consistently linked to positive outcomes; e.g., Constantino, Arnkoff,

Glass, Ametrano, & Smith, 2011). Ahmed and colleagues (2010) found that clients who went on to be optimistic about being able to benefit from treatment after the first session of therapy had therapists who managed to stay understanding, affirming, and supportive during moments of client resistance. In contrast, those clients who went on to be pessimistic had therapists who either attempted to control them ("See things my way") or dismissed their concerns ("Do whatever you want—it doesn't matter to me") at these times. Accordingly, the clients who went on to be pessimistic about treatment, despite not differing from the optimistic clients in their expectations for treatment helpfulness prior to the session, detached themselves from the therapist much more often (disregarding the therapist or doing the opposite of what the therapist wanted). In short, attempts to control and influence during resistance tend to alienate the client and may lower his or her enthusiasm about treatment, while efforts to understand and hear client doubts and concerns do the opposite.

Thus, honing one's skill at systematically listening for and attending to information about client readiness is an important prerequisite for responding flexibly to minimize resistance and maximize the probability of client movement toward change.

Therapist attempts to control and influence the client during resistance alienate him or her; understanding and listening to client doubts do the opposite.

OBSERVING READINESS

Observing Resistance in the Process

One important way resistance can be expressed is interpersonally, through opposition to therapist direction or therapist demands. You make a suggestion, and the client responds with silence, lack of enthusiasm, or "Yes, but . . ." or "I can't." You ask a question or make a reflection, and the client interrupts you, ignores it, and follows his or her own agenda. You suggest an alternative way of viewing things or behaving, and the client disagrees. Newman (1994) identifies some common manifestations of ambivalence or resistance in the context of CBT, for example, including limited compliance with or refusal to follow through with homework, taking actions that run counter to what was agreed upon in session, high levels of expressed emotion toward the therapist, in-session avoidance such as silence or frequent use of "I don't know," debates with the therapist, and challenging or disagreeing with therapist comments. Each of these examples reflects resistance that is stimulated or created by the presence of therapist direction or demands.

In essence, these moments reflect how well the two of you are working together (collaborating), and a high frequency of these instances signals that there is disharmony in the working relationship that the therapist needs to correct. As Miller and Rollnick (2002) observe, the presence of resistance in the relationship should operate as a type of "stop signal" indicating that the therapist is working ahead of the client's level of readiness, placing demands on the client (to do, be, or think something) that he or she is not ready for. That is, client resistance to therapist demands offers critical information and represents the client's efforts to protect his or her autonomy and reassert freedom of choice. The onus is on the therapist to be attentive to and hear such messages in order to reestablish collaboration and harmony in the relationship.

In other words, in observing the client's moment-to-moment engagement with the process, you can continually ask, "Is the client moving toward me or away from me?" If you feel you are "not together" and the client is not responding to your contributions and efforts to guide the process, this is a very important signal that you need to work to reestablish client engagement. And a number of different observational systems have been developed to assess resistance in psychotherapy. For example, in their work on identifying ruptures in the therapeutic alliance (a complex interpersonal process between a patient and the therapist that is often subjectively experienced as tension within the therapeutic relationship), Safran and Muran (e.g., Safran & Muran, 1996; Safran, Muran, Samstag, & Stevens, 2002) identify three categories of rupture markers. These include physical behaviors (e.g., averting one's gaze or looking down, turning one's body away, crossing arms), narrative manner or tone (e.g., a long silence, a refusal to respond or minimal response, changing the topic, a demanding or emphatic tone, the use of sarcasm or a mocking tone, interrupting), and narrative content (intellectualization, a vague or abstract narrative, self-justifying statements, helpless behavior, criticism of the therapist, questions about the relevance of interventions or treatment tasks, doubts about being in therapy).

Of the various systems for observing resistance in process, the Client Resistance Code (CRC; Chamberlain et al., 1985; Chamberlain, Patterson, Reid, Kavanagh, & Forgatch, 1984) is widely used and not tied to a particular therapy approach. Thus, it seems more suited to the purpose of identifying client behaviors reflecting resistance across different ways of conducting therapy. Resistance in the CRC is defined as any behavior that opposes, blocks, diverts, or impedes the direction set by the therapist. The CRC consists of multiple categories of resistant behavior. These are summarized in Table 3.1. Note that resistance in process (opposition to the therapist) can be expressed either verbally (e.g., "I can't" or "I won't") or nonverbally (e.g., by ignoring or withdrawing).

TABLE 3.1. Types of Resistance Defined in the Client Resistance Code

Confront/challenge/disagree. Here, the client's remarks indicate dissatisfaction with the therapy and/or the therapist and/or disagreements with the therapist. This may also include noncompliance with a session directive or suggestion by the therapist.

Hopeless/blame/complain. These statements indicate an inability of the client to change. They include remarks of an "I can't" nature, for example, "I can't because I don't have it in me" or "I can't because I don't think anything will help." They also include statements of prolonged, repetitive, defeatist, or negative conditions; hopelessness and self-blaming remarks; blaming statements that hold others responsible for present, past, and anticipated difficulties; and complaining statements that attribute the source of one's problems to someone else or something else without explicitly blaming that source for it.

Defend self. This involves defending, justifying, making excuses—for example, "I really did mean to do it [e.g., a homework assignment], but I just got too busy at work."

Sidetracking and own agenda. Here, the client talks about other things in response to therapist attempts to focus the client on his or her problems and working on them. This includes client statements indicating a desire to talk about issues that are different from the current direction of the therapist, or client persistence in discussing other related issues. This also includes not attending to the therapist, such as ignoring, or a response from the client that is off the topic of the discussion.

Not responding/not answering/withdrawing. This involves responding to a question or, in response to a direct question, the client is evasive, nondirect, or leaves the statement open-ended.

Disqualify. This involves contradicting an earlier statement made by the client, but not an immediate and/or trivial correction of fact.

If you watch the process of therapy closely, the therapist is typically setting a direction and asking the client to follow, whether it be asking a question, making a suggestion, providing information, or offering a reflection or interpretation. In this sense, in a typical therapy session the therapist is nearly always asking the client to follow his or her lead (e.g., by answering the question, considering the suggestion or information, elaborating on a reflection). Even when being primarily empathic, the therapist is inviting the client (albeit with support for autonomy) to pay attention to and respond to his or her reflection or last statement. The therapist selects something out of what the client has said, puts it into words, and 'asks' the client to respond to this restatement or elaboration. Knowing that the therapist is always issuing such invitations to follow, it becomes possible to discern whether the client is following (i.e., accepting the invitation) or not following the therapist (opposing, ignoring).

Clinical Example 1

Let's contextualize this by illustrating how observations using the CRC can be made in two clinical examples of therapist–client interactions in therapy sessions. In the first instance, the client is discussing her fears about an important upcoming job interview, and the therapist is attempting to help her reframe this experience in order to reduce her anxiety. [Instances of resistance appear within brackets.]

> THERAPIST: Let's say hypothetically that you are on the way to the interview. And instead of saying "Oh my god, I'm going to screw up," let's say you were thinking, "You know what, I already have a job . . . "
>
> CLIENT: [Interrupts.] I try to think that, but I really want this one!
>
> THERAPIST: That's so important. Right. *(slight pause)* But let's say you were thinking "I already have evidence that I do well on interviews 'cause I already have this other job. And I'll just go in there and do my best. So, even though my answers won't be perfect, they'll be adequate." If you were to shift your thoughts like that, how do you think you'd be feeling? Would you be as nervous?
>
> CLIENT: *(softly)* Probably not. [withdrawing]
>
> THERAPIST: Right. You probably wouldn't be as nervous. And what about all these bodily sensations?
>
> CLIENT: *(softly)* Yeah, same. [withdrawing]
>
> THERAPIST: Right. You wouldn't feel so tense. And it would probably be easier to smile and be yourself.
>
> CLIENT: *(softly)* Right. [withdrawing]
>
> THERAPIST: So, the situation is the same, but, depending on how you think about the situation, it really affects all these other areas as well.
>
> CLIENT: *(hesitantly)* Uh huh. [withdrawing] I think I understand that, but when it comes down to it at the time, I don't think of that. All I think about is that I want this job. It's hard to catch myself and stop it. [defending self; hopelessness/complaining; disqualifying]
>
> THERAPIST: Well that's why we're here!
>
> CLIENT: *(dismissively)* Right. [withdrawing]

Many specific instances of client opposition to the therapist can be observed in this brief example. Overall, the interaction contains a feeling of tension and disharmony (noncollaboration or working at cross-purposes). The client is not moving toward the therapist but away from him. Overall, the client is protesting, and this is in direct response to the therapist's repeated attempts to influence her, in this case by making suggestions that the client is not ready to implement. The therapist's questions are also not received as evocative attempts to explore but rather interpreted (correctly) by the client as further demands or attempts to influence (i.e., leading questions or questions with an agenda). The therapist also makes a very brief attempt to hear the client (e.g., "[getting this job] is so important. Right."), but it's not enough to make the client feel that her position and feelings on this subject are understood by the therapist. The effort to understand is also not consistent enough in that it is quickly supplanted (and undermined) by further attempts to persuade the client to the therapist's way of thinking.

The client's withdrawal, passivity in the interaction, and complaints about her inability to do what the therapist suggests are not attempts to irritate the therapist but rather to tell the therapist that his timing is off. They are efforts to communicate a vitally important message, namely, that the therapist is pushing her beyond what she is currently ready for and willing to do. When the client's withdrawal fails to effectively communicate her lack of agreement and unwillingness to go along with the therapist, she more openly discloses her position and protest ("It's hard to catch myself and stop it," which likely means "It's *too* hard to catch myself . . . " or "I don't feel able to catch myself . . . "). When the client says this, she is not asking the therapist to talk her out of feeling that way, but rather asking the therapist to hear, acknowledge, and register her doubts. Unfortunately, in this instance this effort by the client also proves futile in registering her protest in the mind of the therapist.

Clinical Example 2

Let's consider another instance of resistance in the process of therapy to further illustrate how the client's readiness messages can be observed in the ongoing interaction. This client is a college student who worries about being late. Here, the therapist is attempting to help the client by moving her to a less anxiety-provoking perspective on lateness.

THERAPIST: So, even if a person was late once in a while, that's no good?

CLIENT: (*pause*) I don't know. [challenging/disagreeing] Maybe one class in a semester. Things happen right (*physically restless*). But

I don't know (*pause*). [withdrawing] I guess that's the way I see it. [challenging/disagreeing; defending self]

THERAPIST: And does everyone else see it that way?

CLIENT: (*sarcastically*) It doesn't seem like it. People come in late all the time.

THERAPIST: And does it affect their grades or . . .?

CLIENT: But it's disruptive too! . . . you know. [interrupting; ignoring; challenging/disagreeing]

THERAPIST: Sure it is. I'm not saying being late is a good thing. But is it that bad that you would spend time and energy worrying about it?

CLIENT: (*very silently and quickly*) Hmm. [withdrawing]

THERAPIST: So, it's kind of weighing the pros and the cons.

CLIENT: (*very silently and quickly*) Hmm. [withdrawing]

Here the client uses a variety of different strategies (overt and covert) to communicate her unwillingness to go along with the therapist, including interrupting, ignoring, disagreeing and defending her position, and, ultimately, passively withdrawing. These examples also illustrate how immediately responsive the interaction is to therapist demands when made in the context of the client's low readiness for change. Therapist directiveness in this context can very quickly and reliably elicit client resistance. Continually watching for such behaviors thus provides an immediate and readily available source of feedback to the therapist about the client's level of readiness for change. Also, if you find yourself working hard to convince and persuade the client to a different way of thinking or acting (as in these examples), it is also a good sign that the client is not ready to consider such alternatives.

Developing the capacity to decode and hear these important interpersonal messages and respond in a manner that makes it clear that you have heard, appreciate, and accept the client's position is important to reestablishing harmony in the relationship. Failure to do so (and therefore perpetuating resistance) may have important interpersonal consequences that may ultimately disrupt good treatment outcomes. These can include undermining client safety in self-expression and self-assertion, communicating the therapist's lack of acceptance of positions that deviate from his or her own, or undermining the therapist's unconditional positive regard (i.e., "I'll only like or accept you if you agree with me—go along with me").

> *Continually watch for behaviors reflecting resistance.*

Moreover, it is important for the therapist to avoid interpreting client opposition pejoratively as obstructive. Here, the therapist also needs to be alert for feelings in themselves of irritation or anger, which may signal the presence of such negative interpretations. Rather, the therapist needs to work to retain and cultivate the MI spirit (discussed in Chapter 2), including practicing acceptance, prizing, understanding, and preserving client autonomy. This can be particularly challenging in the presence of client resistance to the therapist, in part because these behaviors can be interpreted as thwarting the therapist's well-intentioned efforts to be helpful, and may trigger doubts about one's competence, skill, and influence as a therapist (ultimately leading to defensive efforts to reestablish control).

Infusing MI spirit and methods into treatment, however, can inform the spirit and manner in which therapist inputs and expertise are offered, increasing the probability of client receptivity to them. Such skills, which emerge from the MI spirit or attitude of the therapist, include sensitivity to the timing of suggestions (in terms of client readiness), explicitly preserving client autonomy and authority, and reinforcing the client's freedom to reject and/or adapt therapist inputs (see Chapters 9 and 10). Moreover, a major contribution of MI is that it offers effective means of defusing, responding to, and working with (rather than against) client resistance. These means include specific MI strategies for rolling with resistance that occurs in the therapy process and understanding and positively reframing resistance to change (see Chapters 6 and 12).

Observing Resistance in Client Speech

In addition to observing client readiness in process or interpersonal interactions, important information about readiness can also be gleaned from attending carefully to the client's speech, or how the client talks about change. In fact, a number of studies have supported the importance of being attentive and responsive to client language and utterances regarding change (reviewed by Miller & Rose, 2009). Specifically, expressions of desire, ability, and the reasons and need for change have been found to precede statements of commitment to change, which in turn have been found to predict behavior change. Thus, learning to listen for how clients talk about change (or not changing) is an important prerequisite for shaping effective therapist responses.

First, the client might indicate his or her ambivalence about change directly by expressing a need to change and immediately expressing reluctance to change or the reasons not to do so. The two statements are in opposition and usually occur in close proximity to each other. These statements capture conflict, struggle, or simultaneously competing motives of approach and avoidance. Often, in the case of resisting change, a client offers a reason or incentive to change and then quickly disqualifies or negates it. Such statements often take the following forms:

- "I know I should, but . . . " *(e.g., "I know I should forgive myself, but I just can't").*
- "I want to, but . . . " *(e.g., I want to be happy, but I feel guilty—like I don't deserve it").*
- "I know it doesn't make sense, but I can't seem to stop" *(e.g., "I know worry doesn't help, but I feel like I have to do it").*
- "That all makes sense [or I know these alternative thoughts are true], but I don't believe it." *(e.g., "I know everyone makes mistakes, but I feel like I shouldn't or like I can't").*
- "Logically I know it, but emotionally . . ." *(e.g., "I know I'm not worthless, but it feels like I am").*
- "I should want to do that, but . . . " *(e.g., "I know I should want to leave him because he treats me terribly, but he's not all bad").*
- "I know it would be good for me, but . . . " *(e.g., "I know I would feel better if I got out more, but I just don't feel like it").*
- "Even though I don't want to, it feels like I have to . . . " *(e.g., "I know I shouldn't wash my hands so much, but I can't seem to stop").*
- "I want to believe it, but I can't" *(e.g., "People tell me I am a good person, but I don't believe it").*
- "On the one hand, . . . on the other hand" *(e.g., "On the one hand, I know I should be more assertive, but on the other hand, I worry that others will react badly").*

Second, a high frequency of counterchange talk or statements reflecting arguments against change (referred to as "sustain talk") is an important indicator of ambivalence and resistance to change. These statements include both arguments in favor of maintaining the status quo (e.g., "Worrying helps me feel prepared," or "I'm less anxious if I avoid others," or "I just feel too anxious if I don't check") and arguments against change (e.g., "It would be too hard for me to change," or "I'm afraid of what would happen if I didn't check the stove"). Statements can reflect low desire, ability, or reasons, for needing to change. They can also include low commitment to change (e.g., "I hope to change," or "I'll try") and the absence of taking steps toward change.

> *Persistent sustain talk indicates resistance to change.*

Clinical Example of Sustain Talk

Consider the following clinical illustration, which contains numerous counterchange statements (specific types of client speech about change are notated in brackets). Here, the client is discussing an incident at work with his colleagues about which he was very stressed and worried a great deal. He noted that the incident was resolved and credited his worrying with much of this positive outcome.

> CLIENT: Part of the reason things turn around is because I do worry and I think about what I could do. So, I had all these ideas to make things better [reasons and need to worry]. So, I always find it hard. Sometimes I think, "Well, did I worry needlessly" [reasons and desire for change]? But as I'm worrying, I'm coming up with the strategic alternatives on how to approach something. I think maybe it's because I worried so much that they changed their attitude. If I had been the callous sort of person who said "Well, that's the way it is" and not worried about it, maybe it would have been a more stressful situation [reasons and need to worry].

Later in the interaction the client goes on to elaborate other benefits to worry and reasons against change.

> CLIENT: I'm not so sure that I could worry less because I also think I am a little bit lazy [low ability to change]. I might not give something some thought until I got worried about it [reasons and need to worry]. Without that, I'd be too lazy to think about it ahead of time [low desire for change]. It could be that there's a bit of the worry that gets me going on things [reasons and need to worry]. Because sometimes I wonder if I had nothing to worry about—no kids to worry about and no money to worry about—I'm not sure that I wouldn't just lay in bed all day. And now I never lay in bed. So, I think there is something to having things to worry about that makes you a more productive individual by virtue of the fact that you have those things [reasons and need to worry].

Here the client's language reflects strong arguments in favor of not changing (sustain talk), with very few arguments in favor of change and no commitment statements. Moreover, the client views change as dangerous (risking making her a callous and lazy individual), worry and anxiety as very laudable and valuable (coming up with "strategic alternatives"), and consequently argues strongly against the prospect of change. In the presence of a high number of such statements (arguments favoring the status quo and against change), proceeding with an intervention aimed at change is strongly contraindicated and will likely yield much interpersonal resistance (or resistance to the therapist) and more counterchange talk. In that case, it is best to work from where the client is in terms of readiness and to use MI skills for more fully understanding the client's position, thereby ultimately building resolve for change (addressed in Part III of this book).

Clinical Example of Change Talk

Contrast the foregoing example with an excerpt from a client that contains a high number of statements in favor of change. Here, the client responds to a description by the therapist about how they will work together.

> CLIENT: I can see that this will be helpful [ability and desire to change], which I really need because this anxiety has gotten way out of control. It's ruining my life [reasons for change]. I know it won't be easy [reasons to not change], but if I've built up my thinking to be so negative, I can break it down too [ability to change]. I'm going to watch this week to see what else I have blown out of proportion [commitment language, taking steps].

In this case, careful observation of client statements reveals a preponderance of arguments favoring change, a general optimism about the prospect of change and accomplishing change, and a statement of one's commitment to taking specific actions. In the presence of this resolve, the therapist could most productively work with the client not by further building motivation but by helping the client envision, develop, and take active steps to accomplish the changes they desire (see Part IV). Note that what the client says (e.g., "This anxiety is ruining my life" vs. "It bothers me sometimes that I'm anxious") and the manner in which he or she says it (adamantly, more loudly, with greater force, versus casually and with less intensity) also influence the assessment of the strength of the utterances favoring change or the status quo.

Finally, a significant number of client questions about treatment and/ or the therapist's qualifications, particularly if asked spontaneously (i.e., without explicit inquiry by the therapist) may also indicate the presence of reticence or skepticism about treatment. The client may not directly express doubts but rather ask questions that stem from underlying concerns about treatment. Therapists can (correctly) perceive these as conveying a message of skepticism or doubt rather than as straightforward requests for information. Examples might include: "How effective is this therapy?", "How many people have you seen?", "Have you read my file?", or "Have you ever seen someone like me?" At these times, the therapist can experience a pull toward defending him- or herself or an urge to convince or reassure the client with statements like "Yes, I did read your file," "I am qualified," or "There is lots of evidence that CBT does work." In general, therapists should resist defending themselves at these times, since such client questions are often really statements (e.g., "I'm not sure I believe that therapy can help me" or "I'm not sure I trust you") rather than requests for information. Therefore, responding to them to reflect the underlying meaning (e.g., "It sounds like you have some important doubts about whether this treatment is for you or whether I can help you") tends to be more effective than providing factual information.

Other Observations Signaling Readiness for Change

Miller and Rollnick (2002) also provide a useful list of additional "Signs of Readiness for Change" (see Table 3.2). On a broad level, these are indicators that clients have sufficiently resolved ambivalence and are preparing to

---

TABLE 3.2. Signs of Readiness for Change

Decreased resistance. The wind seems to have gone out of the sails of resistance. Dissonance in the counseling relationship diminishes, and resistance decreases.

Decreased discussion about the problem. The client seems to have talked enough about the area of concern. If the client has been asking questions about the problem area, these stop. There is a feeling of at least partial completion, of waiting for the next step.

Resolve. The client appears to have reached some kind of resolution, and may seem more peaceful, relaxed, calm, unburdened, or settled. This can also have a tone of loss, tearfulness, or resignation.

Change talk. Whereas resistance diminishes, change talk increases. The client makes direct change statements reflecting disadvantages of the status quo, advantages of change, optimism about change, and/or intention to change.

Questions about change. The client may begin to ask what he or she could do about the problem, how people change once they decide to, or the like.

Envisioning. The client talks about how life might be after a change. This can be mistaken for resistance, in that looking ahead to change often causes a person to anticipate difficulties if a change were made. Of course, the client may also envision positive outcomes of change.

Experimenting. If the client has had time between sessions, he or she may have begun experimenting with possible change actions since the last session.

Note. Reprinted from Miller and Rollnick (2002, p. 127). Copyright 2002 by The Guilford Press. Reprinted by permission.

take action toward change. Thus, upon observing such behaviors, clinicians are encouraged to shift from exploration and resolution of ambivalence to helping clients prepare for and commit to change.

SUMMARY

Ongoing attentiveness to and observations of the process of therapy can provide valuable information about a client's engagement in therapy and level of readiness to change, and consequently their receptivity to taking action to change. Honing skills at recognizing resistance, on the one hand, and readiness to change, on the other, is an important prerequisite to matching your clinical style (supportive or directive) to the client's level of motivation. Recognizing resistance both in the unfolding of the interaction (i.e., opposition to therapist direction; disharmony) and in client statements and language about change/treatment (change talk and sustain talk) are two important sources of information about client readiness for change.

Such skills in identifying resistance are not necessarily easy to cultivate and can require concerted effort and practice to develop, particularly since resistance can often be subtle rather than overt. I have also noticed that there can be a reluctance to identify resistance (perhaps because, once noticed, one must deal with it—which can be very challenging), with accompanying tendencies to attempt to "explain away" and dismiss it through attributions such as "That's just his personality style" or "She's just anxious." That is, recognition of resistance should not be automatically assumed but rather appears to be a skill to be cultivated. This is consistent with recommendations by resistance researchers, who emphasize the identification of resistance or tensions in the therapeutic relationship as a key clinical skill (e.g., Binder & Strupp, 1997; Safran & Muran, 1996).

4

∞

Asking about Readiness

In addition to observing readiness in the client language and the therapy process, one can also ask about readiness and have the client self-reflect on his or her level of readiness for change. In this chapter, I offer a number of questions or areas of inquiry that can be useful in getting an initial sense of the client's level of motivation upon beginning treatment. I also make suggestions regarding working with client responses to demonstrate openness to hearing ambivalence and communicating willingness to work with reservations about change. These questions are intended to supplement an initial clinical assessment and may elicit specific information relevant to motivation and client ambivalence. Following this, I briefly review self-report measures that attempt to quantify client self-reported motivation for change, either at the beginning of treatment or throughout the process.

INTERVIEW QUESTIONS TO ASSESS MOTIVATION

- *"How are you feeling about being here today?"* I typically start my first session with any client (after going over the limits of confidentiality and other necessary administrative details) with the following: "People often have mixed and sometimes strong feelings, one way or the other, about coming to therapy. How do you feel about being here today?" This simple question serves two main purposes. First, it communicates interest in learning about the current experience of the client. For many individuals, approaching the therapist's door can be an event laden with powerful emotions (e.g., fear, uncertainty, reluctance, hope, relief). Acknowledging, reflecting, normalizing, and validating these feelings facilitates the therapeutic alliance by communicating both interest in the experience of the client and underscoring the potential significance of seeking therapy. Second, it provides an early invitation for the client to freely express his or her feelings about the act of seeking treatment and indicates that the therapist is open to hearing any reservations the client may have about treatment. There is strong evidence that the act of seeking treatment is often fraught with ambivalence. Most sufferers of anxiety and depression do not seek treatment (e.g., Collins, Westra, Dozois, & Burns, 2004), delay seeking treatment (e.g., Christiana et al., 2000), and/or have numerous fears of treatment (e.g., Kushner & Sher, 1991).

Moreover, client responses to this invitation can be highly informative in assessing readiness for change and treatment. If clients articulate mostly or exclusively positive feelings (e.g., "I'm relieved to be here," "I've been looking forward to it"), this can be an early indication of high levels of motivation. Further, asking clients to elaborate on such responses provides an early opportunity to elicit change talk. On the other hand, if clients express anxiety, for example, therapists have an opportunity to learn more about what coming to treatment means for them and to validate and normalize these concerns. And if clients express reservations about treatment, this provides an initial opportunity to learn about the client's ambivalence and to use MI in responding to it. As just one example, consider the following:

THERAPIST: People often have mixed and sometimes strong feelings, one way or the other, about coming to therapy. How do you feel about being here today?

CLIENT: It was hard for me to come, because I don't like this whole therapy thing.

THERAPIST: So, this is pretty significant—being here. It took some doing. If you're willing, can you say more about your feelings about the idea of treatment?

• "What steps have you taken to manage your anxiety/depression?" Clients vary in the effort they have expended to overcome their difficulties with anxiety and related problems prior to entering treatment. For some, coming to therapy is among their first steps, while others have already expended considerable effort in learning about or addressing their problems (e.g., reading self-help books, looking for information on the Internet, engaging in previous counseling, trying exposure or attempting to be more active). Miller and Rollnick (2002) discuss "taking steps" as one positive indicator of client motivation. In general, active efforts to learn about and overcome the problem indicate higher levels of motivation and less ambivalence about change. Engaging in exposure or behavioral activation, for example, is a behavioral marker of resolved ambivalence since approach tendencies are stronger than avoidance motives. Also, if the client has taken specific steps, the therapist can inquire as to what motivated him or her to take these steps (e.g., "Why would you do X? It sounds hard/effortful"), thus learning about important sources of the client's motivation and eliciting change talk.

• *"Have you had counseling before for anxiety/depression?"* If the answer is "No", you can ask what motivated the client to seek treatment now. This inquiry can often elicit important information regarding the client's current incentives and motivations in considering therapy (e.g., "I've just had enough," "It's causing problems at work or with my family"). If the client has had previous counseling, it can be very informative to ask about what that experience was like. You can ask about both the effectiveness of that experience (e.g., "How helpful was it?") and the process (e.g., "What was it about that experience that led to its being helpful or not helpful?").

Previous experience is a very important determinant of expectations and optimism about therapy. Clients who have had previous positive experiences are typically much more eager to reengage with therapy than those who have had negative treatment experiences. In fact, those with negative experiences are likely to have hesitated considerably before reengaging with therapy, and their doubts and concerns need to be openly discussed and acknowledged. They may also require explicit reassurance, based on knowledge of their previous experiences, that therapy will be conducted in a manner befitting their preferences and needs. In either case, it is useful to spend some time becoming knowledgeable about what the client liked and did not like about this experience and what was helpful and not so helpful. This shows both an interest in the client's previous experiences and a desire to learn from these experiences in shaping the therapy.

• *"Often people have specific ideas or preferences about what therapy should look like. If we worked really well together, what exactly would that look like, what would we be doing, what would be happening in our sessions?"* Learning about client preferences for therapy process is important to offering choice in treatment and tailoring the therapy to your client's needs. Some clients express no particular preference (especially those who have not had previous therapy) and merely articulate that they are "open" to suggestions and recommendations. Often, however, clients have particular ideas about what they want or need (particularly since information about therapy is now more widely available than ever), and these ideas might also be based on their knowledge of what has been helpful for themselves or others, such as family or friends. Also, clients often come to therapy only when their other efforts and coping attempts have failed. Thus, they come in with particular experience and opinions about what is needed.

> Ask clients about their preferences in order to tailor their treatment.

Finally, it is important to be responsive to the client's needs and preferences for how therapy should unfold and to tailor your treatment accordingly. A candid discussion about what you can and cannot do is important, especially in those cases where the client's needs may diverge from what you can or are willing to provide. For example, one client I worked with, a married woman with three teenage children, was having extramarital affairs. In response to the question about her vision of therapy, she was adamant that what she needed was practical coping skills to shore up her willpower to resist the extramarital affairs since she did not wish to jeopardize her family. My own belief was that a likely productive focus of therapy would also involve exploring what needs were being met by these infidelities (i.e., what compelled her to have the affairs). Thus, I reflected my understanding of her desires for the focus of treatment but also suggested an additional focus, specifically saying:

> "I hear that your goal is to improve your resolve to stop this behavior and to develop stronger coping strategies to do so. Sometimes, in addition to that, it can be helpful to spend some time exploring what is driving this behavior that you dislike so much. This can be useful in my experience in terms of understanding what the problem is and what leads you to do this so that you can more effectively navigate helpful responses to these urges. However, that may not be of interest to you. What are your thoughts about that?"

In this manner, we were able to negotiate a process that was responsive to her goals while also being true to my beliefs about what would constitute a helpful approach to this situation.

- *"What are your concerns/doubts about therapy?"* Clients who spontaneously (i.e., without an explicit invitation) communicate doubts about you or the therapy are likely quite high in treatment or change ambivalence, in my experience. Most clients, however, may not do so for a variety of reasons, even if they have reservations about change or treatment. Most clients want to "put their best foot forward" regarding their interest in overcoming problems. They may expect (perhaps based on previous experience), that health professionals are primarily interested in why they want to change (i.e., the reasons underlying their desire to change) and less so in the part of them that resists change. Clients may also wish to be consistent in their words and deeds (i.e., being skeptical about treatment may appear to be at odds with the behavior of presenting for treatment).

In addition, clients may be acutely aware of the pain that a problem is causing but less aware—especially in obviously aversive affective states like anxiety and depression—of any functional aspects of the problem (e.g., "Worrying is my way of caring for others." "I'm afraid that if I weren't depressed there would be expectations that I can't meet."). Finally, clients are typically eager to create a good working relationship with you and may fear that expressing reservations and doubts about the therapy will hamper this or negatively affect your willingness to provide treatment. They may understandably fear that opening up the conversation with "I really doubt that you can help me/that this could work/that I can change" or "I'm not sure I can follow through" will convey the wrong tone. Clients typically require explicit permission and encouragement to express treatment- or change-related fears and concerns.

Thus, eliciting and normalizing reservations about treatment and change can be worthwhile in communicating openness to hearing and working with these common concerns.

> *Encourage clients to express change-related fears and concerns.*

ASSESSING THE CLIENT'S NEED FOR AUTONOMY

Client differences in the need for autonomy are an important determinant of their response to directive and less directive interventions (e.g., Beutler, Harwood, et al., 2011; Beutler, Moleiro, et al., 2002a, 2002b). All clients have a need for self-determination (Deci & Ryan, 1985). In general, clients with a strong need for autonomy (and high resistance to being controlled) benefit more from a less directive therapist style and respond with resistance to a more directive approach, while others prefer more structure and direct guidance and are more responsive to a directive approach. Any therapy can be done in a variety of different styles, from more to less directive. In general, more effective CBT therapists have been found to be more evocative, collaborative, encouraging of the client's active participation, and client-centered than less effective therapists, who generally are more compliance-oriented and therapist-centered (Kertes et al., 2010). Thus, while therapists who are more technically focused may work well with clients with higher needs for structure and direct guidance, it is important for these therapists to adapt their style to meet the needs of those clients who are higher in their need for control and tend to oppose direct advice or suggestions.

Thus, determining a client's relative need for control and autonomy in the therapy process is important to adapting and matching one's approach to the needs of the client and maximizing treatment response. This may be accomplished by attending carefully to client responses to the questions about therapy preferences, problem resolution, and previous treatment experiences and integrating this information to inform the therapy approach and therapist style.

Moreover, careful observation of the client is warranted. Clients who are highly verbal and clearly comfortable with the process of self-exploration may require less direct guidance and structure, while those who are less able to engage with this process may require more scaffolding and structure. In addition, carefully attending to client responsiveness (resistance or cooperation) to teaching, instruction, and guidance is important early in therapy. If the client seems curious, interested, receptive, and eager to learn more, this likely indicates that such direct guidance will be fruitful in the therapy. Conversely, if the client expresses considerable doubts and seems reticent (i.e., expresses resistance), this can indicate that the therapy style needs to shift to a more supportive, MI-infused way of working. Finally, Beutler (2002b) suggests that administering the Therapeutic Reactance Scale (Dowd, Milne, & Wise, 1991) may be useful, but he acknowledges that accurate assessment of reactance potential via self-report is difficult.

Integrated Clinical Example

Consider the following example that integrates a number of the suggestions above. This young woman presented for treatment of OCD. Midway through the initial interview, I noticed that she would often provide short responses to questions and reflections. It felt as though she were holding back and reluctant to disclose and engage.

THERAPIST: This may not be accurate at all, but you seem a bit uncomfortable about being here or not quite sure about this process.

CLIENT: Well, I'm the kind of person that doesn't take things at face value. Like, I don't commit until I'm sure of something.

THERAPIST: So, you're a very discerning person. You're not naive. Before you dive in you really need to evaluate things. And that includes therapy. Good for you!

CLIENT: Yes, I've been in therapy before and it didn't work. So, I'm cautious. I really like to wait and see.

THERAPIST: It makes sense that you would take your time to decide whether to commit. You don't want to find yourself in another unworkable situation. It might be quite helpful to spend some time talking about what didn't work in your previous therapy and what you are looking for specifically now. It's important that we

work in a way that makes sense to you and fits with what you
need. How does that sound?

CLIENT: Good.

In this instance, the client clearly had covert reservations about the
therapy and was scrutinizing the process (and me). By inviting her to verbalize her concerns in a nonjudgmental fashion, this showed attentiveness
to the client's process and exhibited openness to hearing and working with
her reservations. After a discussion of her concerns and her vision and preferences about what a successful treatment process would look like for her,
we collaboratively determined a potentially effective approach and process.
Moreover, I did not assume that this fully resolved the client's reticence
and was also aware that beyond broad discussions of therapy goals and
processes there might also be specific things that I was doing (or not doing)
that could be reducing the client's commitment to therapy. Appreciating
the client's stated wishes to "wait and see," I suggested that we regularly
monitor her progress and that I solicit feedback from her at the end of each
session. For example, at the end of the first session the client was asked:

THERAPIST: So, we decided that it would be good for me to check in
    with you at the end of each session to see what you liked and,
    equally importantly, what you didn't like.

CLIENT: I feel good about it. Again, I don't have a lot of information
    yet, but you seem to have a pretty good grasp of what bothers me.
    I'm comfortable continuing.

THERAPIST: So, overall, so far, so good. At the same time, I'm also
    hearing that some things might be better. [The therapist hears a
    hedging tone in the statement "You seem to have a *pretty good*
    grasp of what bothers me" and invites the client to say more. It is
    also not uncommon for clients to sandwich in criticism with posi-
    tive feedback, as in this example, since critiquing the therapist can
    be difficult for most clients, even when invited to do so.]

CLIENT: Well, sometimes you are a bit too quick to respond. Like, I
    may need more time to think.

THERAPIST: So, I cut you off or pre-empt your thinking process when
    having more time would be more useful.

CLIENT: Yes. I'm often confused about what I think and need more
    time to sort it out.

THERAPIST: I appreciate your willingness to say so. That's really impor-
    tant feedback. I agree with you that good therapy involves having
    enough space to understand and reflect on your own thoughts

and feelings. I will definitely work on being more aware of this and will check back with you regularly in the future to see if I've struck a better balance. Does that sound okay?

CLIENT: Yes. That would be good.

When soliciting reservations and doubts, and particularly when soliciting negative feedback about one's own performance, it is critical that the therapist work toward being able to hear this without being affronted or wounded by it. The therapist needs to effectively communicate both verbally and nonverbally (i.e., in spirit) that he or she is indeed open to hearing these concerns. This can be a difficult but very worthwhile skill to cultivate, since failure to be genuinely receptive to feedback would communicate to clients that it is indeed not safe to be candid, despite being invited to do so. For example, in the scenario above, I was momentarily "cut" by the client's specific critique. My own values incline strongly toward the client's active involvement in the process as a major source of therapy benefit. To hear that I was being experienced as—and indeed was—pre-empting this process was a difficult message to absorb in the moment but was, of course, invaluable feedback. Upon reflection, prior to asking the client about her doubts, I was perceiving that she was reticent about therapy, and thus I was working harder to prove myself worthy of being her therapist. In other words, she was right about my overeagerness! Client critiques do contain truths that we must be willing to hear—however discrepant they are from our preferred self-views. In addition, for some clients, such as those who feel they must always defer to others (e.g., those with social anxiety), the process itself of being invited to give negative feedback and experiencing another as receptive to this without catastrophic consequences is, in and of itself, therapeutic (e.g., reflecting modeling and accepting imperfections).

> Be willing to hear client critiques, as they contain truths.

SELF-REPORT SCALES OF MOTIVATION

A number of self-report measures of motivation for changing anxiety and the related problem of depression have been developed. These scales are typically much better predictors of premature termination of therapy than of treatment outcome. Motivation is a broad construct that has been variously defined, and the multiple self-report scales reflect this heterogeneity. In some cases, measures were developed in the substance abuse domain and adapted to the domains of anxiety and depression. This is the case for the most widely used measure of motivation, the University of Rhode Island

Change Assessment. Below several of the more commonly used scales are briefly described, along with two newly developed scales designed to assess ambivalence in these populations and a related measure of outcome expectations.

Since motivation can fluctuate rapidly within a session and even clients with high levels of motivation can experience momentary reluctance to engage with therapy, clinicians would do better to become attuned to markers of in-session ambivalence and resistance (which are discussed in Chapter 3). Nonetheless, there are some contexts (especially research contexts, since observational coding is time-consuming) in which it is desirable to have a scale in which the client reports on his or her own motivation, and a number of these have yielded positive relationships with outcomes in some studies.

University of Rhode Island Change Assessment Scale

The University of Rhode Island Change Assessment Scale (URICA; McConnaughy, Prochaska, & Velicer, 1983) was developed by Prochaska and colleagues to capture the various stages of change in their transtheoretical model (TTM; Prochaska, 1999). It was intended to be applicable to a broad range of problems. According to the TTM, change progresses through five stages: precontemplation (not yet considering change); contemplation (actively considering change but ambivalent); preparation for change; action (deciding to make changes and actively working toward this); and maintenance (having changed and working on consolidating the change and preventing relapse). The URICA consists of 32 items representing four stages of change in the TTM, with eight items for each of the precontemplation, contemplation, action, and maintenance subscales. Profiles of scores are often used to identify the individual's readiness for change.

Research using the URICA has been extensive (for a review, see Prochaska & Norcross, 2004), with populations including substance abuse, health-related behaviors such as smoking and weight loss, as well as more traditional psychotherapy populations such as those with anxiety disorders. In general, the URICA appears to be a better predictor of treatment dropout than outcome. Results are equivocal in terms of the URICA's ability to predict outcome, with some studies providing supportive evidence and many other studies failing to find support (for reviews, see Littell & Girvin, 2002; Sutton, 2001; Wilson & Schlam, 2004). Reviews of research on the TTM have identified a number of other problems, including marked inconsistency in terms of which stage predicts dropout or treatment-induced change, inconsistencies in the definition of stages, the failure of participants to fit neatly into one of the stages, and the lack of support for sequential movement through the stages.

Client Motivation for Therapy Scale

The Client Motivation for Therapy Scale (CMOTS; Pelletier, Tuson, & Haddad, 1997) is a 24-item measure of client motivation for therapy based on the self-determination theory of Deci and Ryan (1985) that postulates six different types of motivation falling on a continuum of autonomy. In ascending order from least to most intrinsic sources of motivation, they are amotivation, four types of extrinsic motivation (external, introjected, identified, and integrated regulation), and intrinsic motivation. The CMOTS yields subscale scores for each type of motivation. After initial scale development, Pelletier (1997) gave the CMOTS to 140 clients receiving therapy from various therapists in the community. They found that the scale had good internal consistency, conformed to the theoretically derived factor structure, and possessed good convergent and discriminant validity. For example, higher levels of self-determination were correlated with higher ratings of the therapist as supporting autonomy, while lower levels were associated with the perception of a more controlling climate in therapy. Zuroff et al. (2007) reported that high scores on the CMOTS were associated with increased rates of short- and long-term improvement in three different types of psychotherapy for depression. And Westra and colleagues (2009) found that clients with GAD of high severity reported greater increases in intrinsic motivation with MI pretreatment, compared to those of high severity receiving no pretreatment. However, the Westra et al. study failed to find support for the capacity of the CMOTS to predict treatment outcome in CBT for GAD. Thus, while demonstrating some promise, the CMOTS requires further research to support its utility.

Nijmegen Motivation List 2

The Nijmegen Motivaton List 2 (NML2; Keijsers, Schaap, Hoogduin, Hoogsteynes, & de Kemp, 1999) was designed to be administered in the early phase of CBT. It consists of 34 statements that are rated by clients according to the extent that each applies to them. While several studies have supported the ability of the original 12-item scale to predict treatment outcome in CBT for anxiety (de Haan et al., 1997; Keijsers, Hoogduin, & Schaap, 1994a, 1994b), it was found to have weak psychometric properties. The NML2 has stronger psychometric support than the original scale with adequate internal consistency and test–retest reliability (Keijsers et al., 1999). The NML2 has three factor analytically derived subscales that include preparedness (intent to actively participate), distress, and doubt (reservations about treatment or treatment benefit). There is limited support for the utility of the scale in predicting dropout or treatment outcome. For example, the preparedness subscale, but not distress or doubt, has been found to predict treatment dropout and perceived treatment helpfulness in a heterogeneous psychotherapy outpatient sample (Keijsers et al., 1999) and in CBT for panic disorder (Keijsers, Kampman, & Hoogduin, 2001). And the scale also failed to predict outcome in CBT for panic disorder (Kampman, Keijsers, Hoogduin, & Hendriks, 2008; Ramnero & Ost, 2004).

Willingness Scale

The original version of the Willingness Scale (WS; Burns, Shaw, & Crocker, 1987) asks respondents how willing they would be to try each of 45 activities to overcome feelings of depression if it were suggested by a therapist or trusted friend. Previous research with depressed outpatients supports the construct and predictive validity of the WS (Burns et al., 1987; Burns & Nolen-Hoeksema, 1991; Burns & Spangler, 2000). The revised, short form of the WS asks respondents whether they would be willing to try each of nine coping activities, such as "Try new ways of relating to other people," "Get started on a task I've been putting off," and "Confront my fears, even if it makes me anxious" (Burns, Westra, & Trockel, 2010). Response options range from "Definitely not" (0) to "Extremely willing" (4). The revised WS has been found to have high internal consistency and predictive validity. For example, using structural equation modeling, scores on the revised, short form of the WS were found to have strong causal effects on changes in depression, even over a brief course of inpatient treatment (Burns, Westra, & Trockel, 2010). And higher willingness has been found to partially account for the relationship between homework compliance and reduced symptom severity in outpatient CBT for depression (Neimeyer, Kazantzis, Kassler, Baker, & Fletcher, 2008). While further research is required, early research on the WS suggests that it has promise in the prediction of treatment response in depression.

Ambivalence Questionnaire

The Ambivalence Questionnaire (AQ; Brody, Arkowitz, & Allen, 2008) is a newly developed measure designed to capture ambivalence about behavior change. Respondents list a specific problem they are trying to change, and subsequent questions are answered with reference to that desired change. The AQ consists of 21 statements reflecting reasons for change and reasons against change, respectively. Each item is rated on a 5-point Likert scale according to the degree to which it applies to the respondent. A decisional balance score can be calculated for each participant that takes into account both the overall magnitude of the pro and con ratings and their strength relative to one another. Preliminary studies by Brody et al. (2008) support the concurrent and predictive validity of the AQ. For example, higher scores on the AQ (i.e., less ambivalence) have been found to be associated with greater reductions in their body mass index 12 weeks later among those attempting self-directed weight loss.

Treatment Ambivalence Questionnaire

The Treatment Ambivalence Questionnaire (TAQ; Rowa, Gifford, McCabe, Antony, & Purdon, 2010) is a newly developed 30-item self-report measure of concerns about engaging in an exposure-based treatment. A preliminary study by Rowa et al. (2010) found that the TAQ is a reliable measure with three subscales derived from exploratory factor analysis. Subscales measure (1) fears of the personal consequences of engaging in treatment (e.g., personality change), (2) fears of negative or adverse reactions to treatment (e.g., not getting better), and (3) concerns about the inconvenience of engaging in treatment (e.g., treatment is time-consuming). Scores on the TAQ have been found to not simply represent general symptom severity or distress (Rowa et al., 2010).

Change Questionnaire

The Change Questionnaire (CQ; Miller & Johnson, 2008) is a recently developed 12-item measure derived from psycholinguistic research on natural language used by clients to describe their own motivation (Amrhein et al., 2003). First, the respondent identifies what he or she is considering changing, and items are completed with reference to that change. Two items each represent desire, ability, reasons, need, commitment to change, as well as taking steps to change and are rated on a 0 (definitely not) to 10 (definitely) scale according to the degree that each statement describes the respondent's motivation (e.g., I want to worry less, I could worry less, etc.). It can also be adapted to a 3-item version (Importance: It is important for me to . . . ; Confidence: I could . . . ; and Commitment: I am trying to . . .), making it highly amenable to administration in clinical practice. Higher scores indicate higher levels of change talk or motivation. The CQ has good internal consistency and test–retest reliability (Miller & Johnson, 2008). Although the CQ has only been evaluated with an anxiety population in one study (Westra, 2011), this study found that it outperformed the CMOTS in significantly predicting posttreatment and even 1-year posttreatment worry scores among those with GAD.

OUTCOME EXPECTATIONS

Outcome expectations (i.e., the degree of expected improvement in treatment) and motivation for change are different but somewhat overlapping constructs. For example, Miller and Rollnick (2002) identify low optimism about change as an indication for the use of MI and improvements in optimism as an indication for shifting to more action-based treatments. The positive link between higher early treatment outcome expectations and both adaptive treatment process and outcome has been established across numerous studies for various treatments and conditions (for reviews, see Constantino et al., 2011; Greenberg, Constantino, & Bruce, 2005). Thus, if you want to know how well your clients will fare in your treatment, ask them.

Expectations are self-fulfilling and tend to generate the expected response (Kirsch, 1990). Moreover, taking action to alleviate negative affect may be futile in the absence of sufficient expectation that these efforts will be beneficial (for anxiety, Ahmed & Westra, 2009; for depression, Catanzaro & Mearns, 1999). For example, those with greater belief in their ability to manage negative affect effectively not only tend to do so more often, but also the impact of their efforts is more likely to be successful in actual affect regulation as compared to those lacking confidence in these efforts (Catanzaro & Mearns, 1999).

The most widely used scale for assessing outcome expectations is the Credibility and Expectancy Questionnaire (CEQ; Devilly & Borkovec, 2000). It has two subscales that assess treatment credibility (i.e., the extent to which clients believe that the treatment will be appropriate and helpful in the reduction of their symptoms) and client expectancy for improvement in treatment, respectively. The three credibility and three expectancy items are rated on a 9-point Likert scale. Both credibility and expectancy have been found to predict adaptive treatment processes and outcomes (e.g., Borkovec, Newman, Pincus, & Lytle, 2002; Safren, Heimberg, & Juster, 1997). However, investigators have argued that these may not be distinct constructs since outcome expectations may develop at least in part from the credibility of the treatment to the client (Greenberg et al., 2005).

The single outcome expectancy item of the CEQ, anticipated improvement by the end of treatment from 0 to 100%, is reliably predictive of outcome across multiple studies and populations including anxiety disorders (e.g., Borkovec et al., 2002; Constantino, Arnow, Blasey, & Agras, 2005; Price, Anderson, Henrich, & Rothbaum, 2008; Vogel, Hansen, Stiles, & Gotestam, 2006). Moreover, those anticipating less than 70% improvement on this item after the first session in CBT for GAD, have been found to lower their outcome expectations to a far greater extent in the presence of problems in the therapeutic relationship and are significantly less likely to recover their expectations following an alliance rupture as compared to those with initial anticipated improvement of 70% or more (Westra, Constantino, & Aviram, 2011).

Moreover, this single item is especially amendable for use in clinical practice since it enables rapid evaluations of a client's optimism about treatment benefit. Given the ease of administration, the item can be repeatedly administered over the

> *Ask your client, "How much do you expect to improve?"*

course of treatment to capture improvements or declines in client optimism about treatment progress.

SUMMARY

A number of questions to help assess motivation during the initial interview or initial sessions with a client were offered, including asking about past treatment and self-management efforts, doubts about therapy, preferred ways of working together, and immediate feelings about coming in for therapy. One should also observe the client's need for autonomy. Such inquiries demonstrate the therapist's interest in exploring the important topic of ambivalence about change and provide early opportunities to demonstrate openness to processing client feelings and concerns about treatment. A number of self-report measures of motivation in the areas of anxiety and depression were also briefly described.

In general, self-report scales of motivation for change in the domains of anxiety and depression have been more consistently predictive of treatment dropout than treatment outcome. Moreover, self-reported motivation may be sensitive to response or self-presentation bias and prone to ceiling effects, and this may be particularly the case in the domains of anxiety and depression. That is, without guidance and a safe therapeutic environment, it can be difficult for many clients to envision possible "benefits" or reasons to be depressed or anxious. Contrast this situation with findings in the eating disorders domain, for example, where self-report measures of motivation are consistently predictive of treatment outcome and recovery (e.g., Geller, Drab-Hudson, Whisenhunt, & Srikameswaran, 2004; McHugh, 2007; Treasure et al., 1999). It may be much more acceptable to indicate that dieting and watching one's weight are desirable than to report that inherently aversive affective states such as anxiety and depression can have benefits. Thus, developing reliably predictive measures of motivation for anxiety and depression may be particularly challenging.

Although some self-report measures of motivation for anxiety and depression show some promise, and research is continuing to evaluate the utility of new measures, at this stage it may be more clinically useful to include questions relevant to motivation, assess outcome expectations, and rely on the observation of in-session resistance, readiness, and ambivalence. Moreover, resistance observed in-session predicts outcome better than self-reported motivation (Westra, 2011).

PART III

❧

Understanding Ambivalence and Building Resolve

5

❧

Introduction to Working with Ambivalence

The word *ambivalence* derives from the Latin *ambi*, or "on both sides," and *valentia*, or "vigor," reflecting strong feelings, beliefs, or motivations in opposition. The chapters in this part of the book describe specific MI strategies, with clinical illustrations, for understanding and working with client ambivalence about change in order to build resolve and momentum for considering and ultimately taking action to change. If, based on your assessment and observations (see Part II), the client appears to be "stuck," the use of the approach and methods outlined in this section is indicated. This stuckness is generally reflected in the presence of many counterchange statements, repeated resistance to suggestions, multiple previously failed treatment efforts, and the like (see Chapters 3 and 4).

The chapters in this part of the book describe the application of MI as traditionally understood and outlined by Miller and Rollnick (2002) to working with clients with anxiety and common related problems of depression. Moreover, since inner conflict and contradictory feelings about change characterize much of clinical work and can frequently emerge (or reemerge) even when clients are actively taking steps to change, developing and refining skills for effectively navigating ambivalence can be an essential element of effective clinical practice.

CONCEPTUALIZING AMBIVALENCE

On a very broad level, ambivalence about change can be thought about as consisting of the benefits of the status quo and the drawbacks to change, on the one hand, versus the downsides of the status quo and the benefits to change, on the other. Thinking of ambivalence in this way can constitute a broad framework that can help guide the exploration of the client's mixed feelings about change. In general, in working with the status quo side, the therapist seeks to help the client understand "What's good about staying the same?", and "What would be bad about change?" In working with the other side, the therapist works to help the client understand "What are the costs of staying the same?" and "What would be good about change?"

Table 5.1 provides a quick reference to guide this exploration for work with clients with anxiety. It is *not* intended to present an exhaustive list of points of inquiry or exploration, nor is it meant to encourage an information-eliciting attitude (i.e., the question-and-answer trap, Miller & Rollnick, 2002), which is inconsistent with the spirit of MI (see Chapter 2). Presenting this table is also not meant to imply that a high degree of structure should be used in working with ambivalence.

While the exploration of ambivalence can be conducted as a specific structured exercise (e.g., having the client write down specific pros and cons), this is generally far less effective, in my experience, since it can interfere with the cultivation of a flexible, free-flowing conversation about change. The exploration of ambivalence is not the linear straightforward process that this table might imply. Typically, clients move back and forth between reasons to change and not to change, and being sufficiently present to capture this fluidity and complexity is an important element of effectively working through client feelings and perspectives on change. However, using some reference points, or a basic framework, to understand and guide the exploration of client views of change can be useful insofar as it promotes explicit recognition, in the therapist's mind, that ambivalence about change is common, expected, and normal. The framework may be useful to the extent that it helps the therapist recognize that considering change is typically fraught with conflict and that decisions regarding change are far from simple and straightforward. Rather, such decisions are complex and multidetermined. The framework is one way of conceptualizing this complexity and can serve as a useful starting point to stimulate identification and deeper contemplation of the critical

> *The exploration of ambivalence as a structured exercise interferes with a flexible, free-flowing conversation about change.*

issues bearing on the decision to change (e.g., fears of change, valued directions).

These possible points of exploration are intended primarily to encourage an attitude of exploration and curiosity. They represent possible *points of entry* to discussing ambivalence, promoting a deeper understanding of conflicting views of change, fears, and values that bear on decisions

TABLE 5.1. Exploring and Understanding Ambivalence about Change

Status quo/remaining the same	Change
"What's good about being the way you are/the problem/the anxiety/ the depression/being anxious/being depressed?"	*What are the costs of staying the same/the problem /the anxiety/being depressed . . . ?"*
"What helps about avoiding/staying home/not socializing/checking/ ritualizing/getting reassurance/being overprotective/worrying/isolating/ planning/ruminating. . . . ?"	*"What hurts you about anxiety/being depressed/staying home/isolating/not being assertive/checking/getting reassurance/ being overprotective/worrying /ruminating/ ritualizing. . . . ?"*
Variants: • "What needs are being met by the problem?" • "To what problem is this a solution?" • "What positive motives and intentions are being expressed by the problem?"	*Variants:* • "What is the most distressing part(s)?" • "How important/significant are these costs?" • "Exactly how or why does that hurt you?" • "Talk from the part of you that is really bothered by this." • "How exactly is it not okay to see yourself this way?" • "If this problem continued, what would that be like . . . how would you feel . . . in 6 months, a year. . . . ?"
"What would be bad about change?"	*"What would be good about change?"*
Variants: • "If you were to worry less/venture away from home/be more active/be less depressed . . . what would be bad about that?" "How would change create its own set of problems or challenges?" "What does the part of you that argues for not changing say?"	*Variants:* • "What would be better if you weren't anxious or depressed anymore?" "What would you really like your life to be like that's different from how it is now?" "How much does this problem fit or not fit with what you really want in life/who you want to be/where you're going?" "If this problem were resolved, what would that be like . . . how would you feel . . . in 6 months, a year . . . ?"

about change. Most importantly, they provide opportunities for the therapist to demonstrate empathic understanding as a catalyst to helping clients achieve deeper self-understanding. That is, the spirit in which the therapist holds the client's responses (i.e., how the therapist responds to the material offered by the client) is critical for building motivation. In particular, the therapist's sense of exploration, curiosity, demonstrations of empathy, willingness to provide validation and affirmation, elaboration, and to raise awareness are all essential. A topical discussion of pros and cons, or compiling lists of reasons for and against change, is superficial and ineffective, in my experience. Rather, the

> *Active and repeated efforts to understand and elaborate the client's beliefs and feelings invites the client to explore his or her own ambivalence.*

therapist's immersion in the process through active and repeated efforts to more fully understand and elaborate the client's views, values, beliefs, and feelings serves as a crucial invitation for the client to more fully explore, understand, and appreciate his or her views on change. Such conversations cannot be scripted but need to evolve, and the suggestions in Table 5.1 can serve as useful jumping-off points for stimulating and nurturing such conversations.

In my experience, material relevant to ambivalence can be difficult for clients to access, articulate, experience, and integrate. Therapists must show patience, support, and encouragement and provide safety and freedom from pressure to change to allow clients to freely explore and understand their ambivalence. This further underscores the importance of MI spirit in initiating inquiries and discussions about ambivalence. It is imperative that the therapist actively nurture and cultivate the underlying spirit of MI, including freedom from pressure to change, trust in the client's self-righting and problem-solving capacity, creating an atmosphere of discovery, and so on. Entering a discussion of ambivalence with a goal of achieving a specific end that is desired by the therapist (even that ambivalence should be resolved) can be problematic and pull the therapist away from being present and attentive to the unfolding process.

Incidentally, developing skill at working with ambivalence beyond the issues of resolving problems with anxiety/depression can also be very useful. While the use of these methods for helping clients increase their resolve for addressing anxiety and related problems is explicitly considered in this book, the ability to work with varying and conflicting positions on other issues encountered in the context of clinical work is a valuable skill. For example, people feel conflicted about many things, such as relationships, career, parenting, or health decisions, to name but a few: "Should I quit my job?," "Should I end this relationship?," "Should I go back to school?," "Should I relocate?," "Should I stop or start taking a medication?," and the like. Offering clients a framework for thinking about and deepening their understanding of such conflicts, helping them make decisions commensurate with a deeper knowledge of their values, and having the skills to help them productively work through ambivalence beyond developing a standard list of pros and cons (that they have likely already tried) can be a valuable asset in one's clinical skill set.

FOCUS OF AMBIVALENCE EXPLORATION

A solid understanding of the client's presenting problems and goals for therapy is needed in productively working with ambivalence. That is, the therapist should be aware of various dimensions of the client's presenting problems (e.g., comorbidities, major problems of concern to the client) and the specific manifestations of the client's problem(s), such as safety behaviors in anxiety (checking, distractions, planning, situational avoidance, etc.) or behavioral deficits in depression (e.g., isolation, unassertiveness, oversleeping, overeating, communication or relationship issues). These can then be brought into the exploration of ambivalence.

The therapist can help the client explore ambivalence more broadly (e.g., "What's good and not so good about staying the same . . . the status quo . . . anxiety . . . depression?") or more specifically (e.g., "What's good and not so good about isolating, worrying, ruminating, not driving, staying in bed, checking, ritualizing, overpreparing, body scanning, planning ahead, being overprotective, keeping busy, distractions?"). These represent different ways of engaging the client in exploring ambivalence. It is typically useful to start with the broader focus and then bring in more specific concerns.

FLEXIBILITY IN RESPONSE
TO MULTIPLE PROBLEMS AND FOCI

Most clients with anxiety and related problems do not have one specific problem that they experience ambivalence about changing but rather multiple problems. These issues are often linked or are associated problems. For example, a common presentation in anxiety is comorbid depression and interpersonal problems (either predating or emerging as a consequence of the anxiety or depression). One client I worked with, for example, was ambivalent about doing exposure exercises for her social avoidance, doing behavioral activation exercises to improve her mood, taking time for herself to improve her self-care, being less self-critical, and being assertive with family members who were taking advantage of her. In this case, as in most cases, there was not one "clear" behavior that needed exploration but rather multiple behaviors. Over time, I had to move flexibly between helping the client explore her ambivalence across these varied dimensions of the problem. For example: "What are the good things about being there 100% for others?," "What are the good things about not taking time for your own interests?," "What are the good things about sleeping a lot?," "What are the good things about avoiding contact with other people?"

It is also not uncommon for a client to move toward taking action to change one problem while remaining ambivalent about others, for example, becoming more active to combat depression but resisting being assertive with important others. Thus, the therapist must recognize that clients can be at differing levels of change for different problems and move flexibly between developing change plans and supporting action in one area while exploring unresolved ambivalence in another. It is also very common in exploring ambivalence for clients to bring in multiple problems or problem behaviors; that is, exploration in one area leads to exploring other areas of difficulty. As just one example, for one client I worked with exploring good things about worry led to a realization of feeling solely responsible for the care of her children. This led her to reflect on how her husband was not sharing caretaking responsibilities and to consider being more assertive with him in this area. Thus, what started out as an exploration of ambivalence about worry moved to centering on ambivalence about expressing her needs more clearly to her husband.

Finally, in the domains of anxiety and related problems such as depression, the treatment targets are often not predominantly or exclusively behavioral or observable (e.g., avoidance, behavioral withdrawal) but rather tend to involve more opaque, less definable targets such as self-criticism, guilt, rumination, poor self-acceptance or emotion regulation, and experiential avoidance (e.g., avoiding the experience of anxiety or low negative affect tolerance). Moreover, the treatment targets can also take time to emerge and/or can shift during treatment, depending on the primary focus of the client's concerns and the evolution of the therapy/treatment conceptualization.

Thus, flexibility in response to changing client needs is required in working well with MI to resolve ambivalence. At all times, the therapist should follow what is "most alive" for, or of greatest interest to, the client as a guide in determining the focus, rather than having an apriori (or therapist-determined) agenda for where to focus the exploration. Significantly greater traction, or clinical mileage, can be accrued by sensitively hearing what is currently on the mind of, or of most interest to, the client, thereby allowing the client to determine the focus. This also requires sensitively shifting to other foci as the conversation unfolds and the client's focus shifts.

Relatedly, working with ambivalence in any given domain is not a linear process; that is, first one side of the ambivalence is examined and then the other. There is a natural ebb and flow in working with ambivalence, since exploration of one side naturally evokes the other side of the ambivalence. That is, as clients consider what helps about the problem, they begin to point out what doesn't help; and, conversely, as they elaborate the reasons to change and change looms closer on the horizon, they reconsider obstacles to change. Thus, the therapist needs to be prepared to move flexibly between both sides of the ambivalence in helping client's to resolve it.

WHERE TO START

The exploration of ambivalence should begin with what is "most alive" for the client (Rice, 1986; Rice & Saperia, 1984). Connecting effectively with clients means hearing the messages that are most salient for them at any given moment. For example, if clients come in expressing a high degree of change talk, the therapist should work to explore, elaborate, and empathically understand the part of the person that wishes to change. Even if the therapist suspects (based on the presence of other markers of ambivalence or stuckness) that the client is significantly ambivalent about change as to preclude taking action, he or she should nonetheless explore what is most salient for the client at precisely that moment (i.e., start where the client is). If the client is also sufficiently resistant to change, as you suspect, undoubtedly opportunities to explore and understand his or her reluctance about change will naturally and spontaneously present themselves during the course of treatment.

The major advantage of reading and following the client (letting him or her lead to the entry points for the conversation about ambivalence) is, of course, that doing so promotes effective collaboration. The client is assured that you are willing to go where he or she leads rather than following your own agenda. When beginning my own practice of MI, I recall several occasions where I was certain that clients harbored substantive resistance to change (e.g., multiple failed previous treatment attempts), and I had "the answer"—empathically exploring resistance to change. However, these conversations failed to take off and even ended badly, with my efforts engendering resistance. Clients could see through my agenda, and in fact they became resistant to my implied (or explicit) message and insistence that they were resistant to change! Thus, the therapist must continually strive to understand the client's (ever-changing) messages on a moment-to-moment basis.

CAVEAT: A DEVIATION FROM MOTIVATIONAL INTERVIEWING AS ORIGINALLY CONCEIVED

As MI has evolved and the mechanisms underlying its effectiveness have largely yet to be determined, various hypotheses have emerged to explain its impact. This has led to somewhat different prescriptions about how MI should be practiced (see Arkowitz, Miller, Westra, & Rollnick, 2008). The way of working with MI outlined and described in this book reflects my own experience in adapting MI to the treatment of anxiety and related problems. It incorporates all the elements of MI (the MI spirit, elaborating change talk, rolling with resistance, etc.) but differs from MI as traditionally conceived in one major respect.

In particular, my own work with MI centers more firmly on exploring and resolving ambivalence. While I fully agree with Miller and Rollnick (2009) that MI is far removed from a simple matter of exploring pros and cons, my own adaptation of MI involves explicit attention to and even active elicitation of *both* sides of the client's ambivalence. From this perspective, MI can be seen as a type of conflict resolution (between competing aspects of the self), and consequently the therapist helps the client explore *both* sides of the client's ambivalence about change, namely, resistance to change and reasons to change. Most significantly, this means that the client is encouraged to voice and fully elaborate counterchange positions and not exclusively or predominantly change positions.

In MI as traditionally conceived, however, this amounts to eliciting "sustain talk" (or talk in the direction of not changing). Accordingly, elaborating such talk in the direction of not changing would be strongly discouraged, given the hypothesized change talk mechanism of MI. Here, people are thought to talk themselves into changing, and, as such, hearing themselves articulate arguments favoring the status quo would be considered countertherapeutic. That is, from the change talk position, when clients argue against change, they are likely to continue on as before. From this perspective, it follows that the counselor should seek to differentially evoke and reinforce change talk and also counsel in a way that minimizes client arguments against change (Miller & Rollnick, 2009; Miller & Rollnick, in press; Miller & Rose, 2009).

From my own perspective, while elaboration of change talk is essential (and specific methods for doing so are outlined and detailed in this book), change talk also often spontaneously and powerfully emerges when a client develops (with the critical aid of the therapist) a more compassionate and understanding view of the part of him or her that resists change. Moreover, when the client begins to make sense of the good reasons to resist change, they can often more powerfully and persuasively argue against their own counterchange position. Finally, as indicated in the next chapter, when exploring the part of the person that argues against change, such conversations should exemplify the spirit of "rolling with resistance", and one should employ all the methods for coming alongside resistance that are so beautifully outlined in MI. From this perspective, exploring resistance to change amounts to rolling with resistance, albeit in a more extended fashion, rather than momentarily doing do in order to bring the conversation back to change talk.

SUMMARY

Understanding that clients often feel torn about change (as we all do) and that there are powerful competing and opposing forces surrounding change is useful in helping clients navigate ambivalence productively rather than getting stuck or frustrated by it. In other words, change is far from a simple matter of recognizing that there are drawbacks to a given behavior and resolving to do away with the old way of being. Given that clients often assume such a unilateral position on change (i.e., that strong desire for change should be sufficient), cultivating an understanding of the complexities and difficulties of change as fraught with conflicting motives and feelings paves the way for clients to appreciate and more productively explore and understand these forces. Such exploration then allows the client to more fully consider decisions about change informed by a more complete understanding of what is given up and what is being gained. I find that even reminding myself of this complexity can be helpful in resisting internal pressures to push the client to take action to change.

In the next three chapters, the components of ambivalence are more fully elaborated, including understanding and reframing resistance to change, evoking and elaborating talk in the direction of change, and bringing these two perspectives on change together through developing discrepancy.

6

❧

Understanding and Reframing
Resistance to Change

It is much easier to work with clients who are motivated to change than ones who are not. In these situations, our efforts can seem very rewarding and satisfying, our input is typically well received, and things progress relatively smoothly. We may also like and enjoy working with these clients to a greater degree than those who resist our efforts to be helpful. It can be particularly challenging to maintain an equally positive and prizing view of and attitude toward clients who resist change. At such times, it is tempting to start judging clients and to see them as deficient in some way, perhaps labeling them as "unmotivated" or "resistant."

When conducting workshops on MI, I ask therapists to picture in their minds several highly resistant clients in their practice and report how they feel when working with these individuals. Clinicians invariably report experiencing (sometimes intensely) feelings of anxiety, confusion, inadequacy, anger, hopelessness, and frustration. Such feelings are natural and understandable since it's very tempting to view resistance to change as an obstacle to progress—something that gets in the way of and thwarts change (and our efforts). Viewing resistance this way naturally leads to efforts to overcome or remediate these obstacles in order to facilitate movement toward change. And indeed resistance to change seems to automatically pull for therapist efforts to correct it (i.e., the "righting reflex"; Miller & Rollnick, 2002).

If you have ever found yourself in such a position (being frustrated by clients who resist your efforts to help them change), you are not alone. Studies have found marked differences in therapist responses to the same person when they show high versus low levels of resistance to change. In one study, counselors interviewed an individual who portrayed a smoker with varying levels of interest in change (Francis et al., 2005). When the person presented as high in resistance to change, counselors were more confrontational, asked more closed questions and fewer open questions, and offered less praise and encouragement, compared to responses to the same person portraying him- or herself as low in resistance to change. Examining actual therapy sessions in CBT for anxiety, Ahmed and colleagues (2010) compared moments in the same session when clients were cooperative to those when the same clients demonstrated resistance in that session (either to the therapist and/or by making counterchange statements). Client resistance was observed to significantly undercut therapist support. At these times, therapists demonstrated substantially lower levels of affirming and understanding, and substantially more attempts to influence or control the client, compared to moments when clients were cooperative. Thus, client resistance seems to strongly pull for less supportive therapist behavior.

Consider the following illustration from the Ahmed et al. (2010) sessions as an example of this pull of resistance for greater therapist control and less support.

CLIENT: . . . I have tried to relax before . . . , every now and again I try doing it, and then I just go, "Oh, this doesn't work."

THERAPIST: Did you immediately learn how to ride a bike?

CLIENT: No.

THERAPIST: Like, you hop on and you probably fell . . .

CLIENT: Mmm-hmm . . . scratches . . .

THERAPIST: And there's gonna be a couple of scratches along the way in terms of learning to do the relaxation.

As this example illustrates, when clients argue against change, there is a pull to correct or remediate this (to persuade the client of the merits of change or the treatment plan). And this pull can be very difficult to resist. In other words, therapists can find it difficult to allow and "hear" such client dismissals of and reservations about change/treatment.

Unfortunately, rather than being more engaged and onboard with the treatment, clients in the Ahmed et al. (2010) study responded to such therapist efforts at control with much lower levels of engagement with the therapist, less self-expression and self-disclosure (they disconnected, withdrew, and didn't continue to explore their concerns about change or the treatment plan). Similar dynamics have been observed in other therapy approaches as well, in the presence of client resistance (e.g., psychodynamic therapy; Binder & Strupp, 1997). And therapist directiveness in the context of client resistance reliably produces further resistance (see Chapter 3 for further elaboration). Directiveness may be helpful in certain contexts, such as when the client is cooperative, but detrimental in the presence of resis-

> *Directiveness works when the client is cooperative but not when resistance and ambivalence are high.*

tance and ambivalence, when supporting the therapeutic alliance becomes especially significant.

I chose to present this example since it can seem familiar to many readers, perhaps because it seems, almost intuitively, to be the "right thing" to do in order to engage clients who show resistance. As Leahy (2001) notes, CBT therapists faced with resistance or noncompliance are typically encouraged to continue to apply standard cognitive-behavioral techniques, and they have been observed to do so (Aspland et al., 2008; Castonguay, Goldfried, Wiser, Raue, & Hayes, 1996).

But when we examine such directive therapist responses to resistance closely for their impact on client engagement in the therapy, it turns out that such efforts are actually counterproductive to the important goal of engaging clients with treatment. This may be because at these times the therapist is (unintentionally) sending a message to clients that he or she is not open to hearing the client's concerns about (or opposition to) the treatment plan or the therapist. The client hears this message, and assumes it is not safe to articulate such disagreements or go against the agenda of change (i.e., to make statements that go against change or the therapist). Therefore, in order to maintain harmony, the client stops expressing his or her reservations or doubts (at least for the time being). Thus, attempting to manage resistance in this manner may appear to "succeed" (e.g., in the illustration above the client appears to "agree" with the therapist's reasoning), but this may represent acquiescence more than resolution. And this is consistent with evidence that clients tend to defer to therapists and generally minimize or hide their negative reactions about therapy and the therapist while remaining overtly cooperative and pleasant (Rennie, 1994; Rhodes, Hill, Thompson, & Elliott, 1994).

RESISTING THE "RIGHTING REFLEX"

When resistance is viewed as a problem, we naturally seek to remediate or eliminate it. The view of resistance to change (and accordingly the approach to it) presented in this chapter is very different. From the perspective of MI, resistance is not viewed as an obstacle to be overcome but rather as a normal and expected part of the vicissitudes of change. Moreover, it contains important (even vital) information that needs to be attended to, heard, understood, and integrated. Resistance to change can reflect fear, uncertainty, learned survival strategies, attempts to support important needs, and adaptive (at least previously) attempts to solve problems. This view or attitude toward resistance flows from the underlying spirit of MI and naturally leads to more supportive therapist behaviors (empathy, validation, etc.) reflecting an openness to hearing the messages contained in resistance.

The MI therapist recognizes the futility of defeating resistance by controlling it, persuading, or counterarguing. Rather, he or she seeks to actively cultivate a positive perception of resistance to change, actively reframing it to extract the positive value in it—to see the wisdom in it. In MI, resistance is regarded as understandable, meaningful, and important. This naturally results in greater efforts to approach, work with, accept, and understand it. When the therapist acts in this way, the client can begin to develop a more complex and compassionate view of the beliefs and behaviors that often frustrate them. That is, when the therapist "rolls with" resistance in this compassionate and accepting manner, it leads to greater self-compassion and acceptance in the client (which is an important goal in and of itself).

The specific skills presented here for understanding and reframing resistance are consistent with the microskills in MI for "rolling with resistance." In short, in MI the therapist works with rather than against resistance to change, which is often referred to as "dancing" rather than "wrestling" with resistance. Such skills include various types of reflection (simple and complex reflection, double-sided reflection, amplified reflection), reframing, emphasizing autonomy, and coming alongside.

In this chapter, the MI skills of rolling with resistance are discussed in the context of building resolve for change among those who are clearly stuck (i.e., those who show high levels of ambivalence and resistance). In Chapter 12, these same skills are discussed and illustrated when resistance emerges (or reemerges) among clients with higher levels of motivation who are working toward actively taking steps to achieve change. Using the distinction introduced in Chapter 3 (namely, resistance in process and resistance to change), this chapter illustrates how the methods of rolling with resistance can be used to work with resistance to change (i.e., clients' statements reflecting movement away from change), and Chapter 12 illustrates how these same skills can be used as well to manage resistance in process (i.e. resistance to the therapist).

EXPLORING AND APPRECIATING
THE GOOD THINGS ABOUT STAYING THE SAME

Often clients can have significant difficulty in exploring the part of themselves that resists change. Asking clients "What's good about being anxious?," "What are the benefits of anxiety?," or "What are the good things about being depressed?" can understandably be met with resistance (if not sensitively constructed and offered with the requisite MI spirit). It is difficult for clients (and even for therapists) to conceive of what might be "helpful" about such inherently aversive conditions.

As I previously mentioned, I think it may be relatively more difficult for clients with anxiety and depression to articulate possible good reasons for the persistence of these aversive conditions as compared to other problems like restricting food intake or drinking, for example. In these latter instances, the reasons to persist with such behaviors may be more obvious or accessible. Thus, inquiring about the good things about anxiety/depression can be met with a lack of response or with resistance (e.g., "There is *nothing* good about it"). Table 6.1 contains a number of suggestions that may be helpful in navigating this temporary obstruction in order to move the exploration of ambivalence forward.

In exploring the benefits of the status quo and the costs to change, the therapist consistently uses empathic listening to genuinely hear the "good things" the client is attempting to express and achieve through the "problem" (and the bad things he or she is trying to avoid by not changing). The possible inquiries presented in Table 5.1 on working with ambivalence (see the left side of the table) can serve as entry points into this exploration and/or can facilitate elaboration whenever resistance to change arises. That is, what appears maladaptive on the surface is often driven by such core needs as the desire for comfort, safety, connection, control, familiarity, success, freedom from aversive experiences or consequences, and the like. The status quo often offers familiarity, predictability, and a sense of control (i.e., *diablos conocidos*, or "the devils I know"), while change and the steps to produce change are fraught with risk, uncertainty, unfamiliarity, discomfort, and ambiguity ("Can I do it?," "Who will I be?," "What if I fail?," "How will others regard me?," etc.).

> *Maladaptive behavior is often driven by such core needs as comfort, safety, control, and success.*

Consistent with a core assumption of Rogers (1965), the therapist practicing MI believes that people are basically striving to live a good, meaningful life, doing the best they can with what they have and what they have learned. Thus, when people act in ways that don't make sense to them (or to others such as family members or helpers), there are "good reasons" underlying these actions and beliefs. One rule of thumb is to assume that *if a client is thinking/doing something and persisting with it despite all his or her efforts not to—there's an important reason(or reasons)*. Clients have been "led astray" by learning history (e.g., the necessary rules for survival

TABLE 6.1. Navigating Resistance to Exploring the Benefits of the Status Quo

Check your MI spirit. Offering anything without the underlying client-centered spirit of MI is problematic and likely to fail to achieve traction. In the case of exploring reasons for the status quo (and reasons to resist change), it is imperative that the therapist work hard to cultivate a nonpejorative understanding of these possibilities and to reframe these often difficult realizations with empathic understanding and validation of the underlying positive intentions and motives of clients (e.g., as satisfying critical, universal needs for connection, safety, comfort, prevention of other problems). Explicitly cultivating (in your own mind) and encouraging a compassionate and open attitude to understanding the powerful forces that inhibit or block change can soften client frustration and self-criticism regarding change. The more the therapist cultivates a patient, accepting, understanding attitude when beginning (and throughout) this exploration, the less likely the client is to resist the exploration.

Provide a rationale. Providing a credible rationale that makes sense to the client is an important component of any intervention, including MI. Communicating your view of the importance and relevance of ambivalence and how exploration of this can be an important component of treatment can increase client receptivity to this way of working. Several points can be communicated, including:

- Ambivalence about change is normal and common. Clients often expect that they shouldn't feel conflicted about change and that change should be unquestionably desirable. However, in undertaking any change, it is only normal to have conflicting feelings and thoughts about it—a tug of war between desiring change, on the one hand, and resisting it, on the other. And the latter often sabotages our best intentions and best-laid plans to change. Clients can feel some relief at having this approach–avoidance dilemma explicitly identified and the emotions accompanying "being stuck" validated— for example, "Sometimes it can be aggravating to "know" what you need to do and yet not see yourself doing it."
- Change is difficult! While change might be desirable, the process of change is not and in fact, is typically quite difficult. Many people falsely assume that change is easy, that they should want to change and readily embrace it. Change can be turbulent and involve a lot of upheaval and losses—some things have to be given up (e.g., old ways of thinking, relating, coping, or being) in order for new ways of being to take their place. As Mark Twain once said, "Everyone likes progress, but no one likes change."
- Therapy offers an important space to explore these different "parts of yourself" that one day insist on change and the next day try to talk you out of it." Exploring these conflicting feelings, these "two minds" about change can help the client be more ready to make change and more prepared to deal with the obstacles that will inevitably arise when they start to do so. Change not only involves taking action; in fact, action is among the last steps in the change process. It also involves planning for change, thinking about change, weighing the pros and cons, becoming more aware of the benefits of change and also the costs of change, and wrestling with conflicting feelings about change. This provides an important opportunity to acknowledge the totality of the client's

(continued)

TABLE 6.1. (*continued*)

experience, namely, an important part of the client that naturally resists change and has important concerns about change that need to be acknowledged, integrated, and understood. This is particularly helpful, in my experience, with clients who exhibit significant frustration with themselves at "knowing" they should change but who nonetheless are unable to do so.

• Reminding clients that "if there were no advantages to staying the same (e.g., being anxious, worrying, avoiding, being unassertive), you would have changed a long time ago. If there were nothing but costs, you wouldn't have the problem anymore," can be helpful. You can encourage the client by stating "Even if the arguments seem ridiculous, try identifying what your anxiety says or argues to get you to conform to what it wants you to do."

Frame the exploration of pros to the status quo as uncovering barriers to change. Framing the exploration as "Exploring what might get in the way of making the change you are clearly interested in making" can be useful in helping clients become more aware of the reasons for the status quo. Understanding these objections to change (or important reasons to resist change) is useful in increasing awareness of the resistance that will inevitably emerge in the change or action-oriented phase of treatment. I recall one client who articulated a high degree of change talk about being less perfectionistic and was adamant that what he needed were practical strategies for achieving this goal. He often had difficulty, however, in implementing the suggestions we developed. I suggested that incorporating a firmer knowledge of the arguments his perfectionism uses to get him to comply with its demands might be useful in increasing the potency and strength of the alternative thoughts and behaviors that he was eager to implement. Framing the exploration in this way, as barriers or saboteurs in implementing action toward his goals, was a productive entry point to helping him explore and more fully integrate the forces in him that resisted change (i.e., argued for the status quo).

Suggest some possible reasons for the status quo. It can also be helpful to prompt the exploration by making a suggestion or two about possible advantages to the status quo (or disadvantages to change). For example: "People commonly tell me that worry helps them to feel in control or prepared. Is that part of it for you?," "Not being assertive with people means less conflict and more harmony. Does that make sense at all for you?," or "A lot of people feel that if they stopped worrying about others, that this would mean they don't care. That may or may not fit for you, though. What are your thoughts?"

Validate the status quo's advantages early in the exploration. It is also important to readily acknowledge and fully validate the identified advantages, particularly early on during the exploration process. This requirement is vital in order to make it safe for clients to articulate the advantages of not changing. That is, people may fear that, if they admit that there is a part of them that doesn't want to change or has good reasons to resist change/treatment, this reluctance will be viewed pejoratively by the therapist or even by themselves. Thus, openmindedness and even receptivity to the articulated benefits of *not changing* is important for the therapist to communicate early on. This enables both the therapist and the client to explore barriers to change in a nonpejorative and nonjudgmental atmosphere.

Regard ambivalence as a process marker. Finally, I have seen others practicing MI (and often have experienced this myself) who productively engage the client in exploring ambivalence by waiting for ambivalence to emerge naturally in the conversation. Rather than setting out to explore or resolve ambivalence, the therapist can patiently wait for these opportunities to spontaneously arise. That is, ambivalence (like resistance) can be thought of as an important process marker that, when it emerges, indicates a need to shift to specific approaches or strategies.[a] This helps the process move more fluidly, be more emergent, and more client- rather than therapist-driven (i.e., more responsive to what the client is working to understand in the moment). When resistance to change emerges in this context, the therapist helps move the exploration of it forward by empathically following and elaborating the material that arises spontaneously for the client in contemplating change.

[a] This is similar to the strategy used in emotion-focused therapy (EFT), in which a defining feature of the approach is that intervention is *marker-guided.* Research has demonstrated that clients enter specific problematic emotional processing states that are identifiable by in-session statements and behaviors that mark underlying affective problems and that these afford opportunities for particular types of effective intervention (Greenberg et al., 1993). EFT therapists are trained to identify the markers of the various types of problematic emotional processing problems and to intervene in specific ways that best suit these problems.

and getting affection/support from important others) and previous experience (e.g., avoiding a threat is reinforcing in that it creates a positive feeling of safety and reinforces the validity of the negative assumption). That is, clients may not yet have learned more adaptive ways of meeting or satisfying these core needs.

Moreover, these underlying positive intentions are things that reflect our common humanity; that is, we can all relate to the need to be connected to others, have others think well of us, be safe, and so on. In using MI, then, the therapist seeks to validate that the ends are highly desirable and basic to human needs. It is the means by which people have learned to achieve those ends (or when those means no longer work) that can become problematic. Thus, the job of the therapist is to *know* that clients are seeking good things, to help clients discover the motivations, needs, and desires that are being expressed through the "problem," and to increase awareness of these so that clients can evaluate for themselves the need for and utility of their assumptions/behavior in light of their underlying values and needs.

Once understood, the meaning of the behavior often becomes clear, as do the reasons why the client would cling to the "problem" and resist relinquishing it. In this exploration, one often has a sense of the problem as "making sense" and the behavior as necessary (or necessary in the absence of broader awareness) to meet important underlying needs. In other words, the "problem" and the client's hesitation about changing always make sense, even though they may not appear to initially, and it is up to the therapist and client together to discover the level on which the current way of being makes sense.

For example, one client I worked with began to realize that his OCD symptoms were closely connected to anxiety about (frequent) interactions with his family. His family was highly intrusive and failed to respect any boundaries the client attempted to set for himself. Through inquiring about the possible "good things" about the OCD, the client discovered that his symptoms allowed him to set important boundaries and do so in a way that the family respected and allowed (e.g., "You can't come to my apartment since I would have to clean excessively afterward" or "If you touch me, it means I'll have to spend hours washing afterward"). Recognizing the "value" of the OCD allowed him to reframe his understanding of it and move away from a pejorative view of it to a more compassionate one. For example, he remarked that "I always perceived my OCD as 'sucking the life' out of me, but now I see that in a weird way it has actually helped me to live my life." This reframing of the problem ultimately helped him to work much more effectively with the OCD, enabling him to gain an important sense of control and choice over the symptoms rather than being a victim of their involuntary appearance.

Or, consider another example of how a problem can have merits as an unrecognized solution to other problems. This client presented with the goal of working on generalized anxiety and a blood/injury phobia. However, we achieved absolutely no traction when using a CBT approach, and homework compliance was virtually absent. When I shifted to MI, the client revealed a larger contextual significance for her remaining anxious. In particular, she reported significant tension with her husband, who was adamantly insisting that they have children. The client had no interest in having children, but she greatly feared expressing this to her husband. Instead, she noted that "I just keep telling him that when my anxiety is better, then we can think about having children." Thus, for this client the anxiety "problem" made sense as a "solution" (however imperfect) to a much larger problem, namely, her fear of communicating openly with her (very dominating) husband and the implications for her marriage of her lack of desire for children.

A very important role for the therapist, then, in my experience, is to know and communicate that the client's "problem" is understandable, given his or her unique experiences, particular circumstances, and ways of construing the world. Linehan (1997) has elaborated the role of validation and has stressed its importance particularly for those with interpersonal problems who have had repeated experiences of invalidation. While empathic listening is itself validating, validation also goes beyond empathy to explicitly communicate an understanding of the wisdom of a response, belief, feeling, or behavior on either a logical or functional level. Statements such as "Of course," "Naturally," "How could it be otherwise?," "That makes so much sense," or "Oh, I see" are common when reflecting the validity of the client's experience. The therapist searches for, communicates, and may even amplify that the client's responses are understandable, reasonable, functional, logical, or fit with learning history or current circumstances (Linehan, 1997).

It can be helpful to have scaffolding for this type of exploration, and to this end a number of prompts for further exploration and unfolding an understanding of resistance to change are presented in Table 6.2. Again, the therapist is attempting to stimulate a free-flowing conversation about resistance and thus, rigid adherence to the possible points of inquiry and elaboration in the table is not recommended. Nonetheless, I have found them useful in stimulating the often difficult task of more fully understanding and appreciating resistance to change. And more broadly, such prompts may be useful in helping the therapist cultivate MI spirit and attitude.

Clinical Examples

Consider the following two clinical examples illustrating the exploration of good things about anxiety. The first is from a session with a married woman with three small children who presented with severe GAD, where health anxiety was a major theme. She came to the session with David Burns's (2006) book *When Panic Attacks* in hand and noted, "While it's kind of helpful, he said you had to be willing to do the exercises and ready to change. I know that I'm not. There is something holding me back from doing this program, even though I tried. I just can't imagine being without the anxiety." The second example involves using MI to explore the advantages of agoraphobic avoidance in a married woman with two small children who had been in treatment, unsuccessfully, on three previous occasions. In each case, the dialogue is annotated with remarks about how the therapist is hearing and responding to the client within the overall framework of working with ambivalence.

EXPLORING GOOD THINGS ABOUT WORRY

THERAPIST: What's good about worrying . . . being on guard about your health? [inviting the client to elaborate on the merits of the status quo position]

CLIENT: I have to be! If I am going to get cancer, then I can catch it early and maybe do something about it.

TABLE 6.2. Prompts for Exploring Resistance to Change

Summarize and link with the value of the behavior/belief. For example: "So, one advantage, if we can call it that, to staying away from people is that you don't risk rejection or disappointment. That sounds really useful, and here you've found a way to reduce feelings that put most of us on our knees."

"And how important is that?" For example: "Is this a minor thing, like 'Oh, by the way, by worrying I get to show people how much I care,' or is it bigger than that?" Or "How important on a scale of 1 to 10 is X [e.g., feeling in control, being comfortable, avoiding rejection]?" Then you might process the response further. For example, if importance is rated 8 out of 10, you can ask, "What goes into that 8? What makes that so important?"

"Tell me more about . . . X [needing to be safe, preventing bad things from happening, ensuring that you don't get rejected, needing to be in control, etc.]."

Link to a common humanity. For example: "I can imagine where you're coming from. If I felt that every time I took at chance at opening myself up to others that I would end up with enormous disappointment and rejection to deal with, I wouldn't be eager to do that either." Or "If I believed that showing weakness would mean that other people would lose respect for me, I don't think I would be keen to advertise my flaws either."

Resonate and prize. For example: "You've got a great strategy here; this is not a problem, this is a solution." Or "If I had a strategy that could keep me safe, prevent disappointment, give me a purpose in life, help me feel connected to others, minimize hassle and frustration, increase my comfort, keep others from thinking negative things, and the like, how much do you think I would use it? People are hungry for these very important things, and this is a way of getting some of those things. It may not be perfect in an ideal world (and might have downsides that we can explore), but it is certainly not without its merits."

"And what has been your experience with the opposite of what the anxiety tells you to do? That is, what has been your experience with not avoiding?" Many clients with anxiety who are stuck have tried to approach the situations they feel a need to avoid and have had negative experiences in doing so (making them reticent about exposure). Here, you could say, "It makes a lot of sense, given your disastrous and painful experiences with trying to be assertive, that you wouldn't want to go there again. You're trying to feel better, not worse." Or "When you describe it, your recent attempts to drive on the highway sound almost traumatic. No wonder you don't want to try it again. It would be like retraumatizing yourself. It would make you more afraid, not less."

Or you could resonate with the nonsensical nature of the "solutions" and advice others have offered (given your understanding of the person's perspective). For example: "So, pleasing other people and thinking about what they want and need gives you a powerful sense of connection to others, an important sense of being needed. And then others come along and say, 'Oh, you should just give that up because it's far better to be assertive.' That's like asking you to give up your purpose in life. I know who will win that argument and who *should* win that argument. It makes sense that you would have no success in doing that because you are after something far more wonderful and fundamental by being there 100% for others."

Using reflection, guess at the client's meaning and underlying beliefs. For example, if a client identifies an advantage of worry as "Worrying about what could happen keeps people safe," you might use reflections to guess at further meaning, such as "So, your thoughts give you a sense of power. The anxiety tells you that they can prevent bad things from happening." Or "It sounds like you're feeling you couldn't handle bad things that might happen." Or if the client notes that "blending in and not standing out prevents others from being critical," you might guess, "It sounds like you're thinking that 'if others reject me it's terrible.' There's no coming back from that." Or "The only way to have people like me is to please them all the time." Or if the person identifies an advantage of worry as "It allows me to feel in control," you might "guess" at the underlying reasons for nonchange, such as "You are concerned that if you don't worry you will spiral out of control."

Explore developmental origins. In my experience, people often spontaneously allude to the developmental origins of the behavior. If the client doesn't do so spontaneously, you can ask, "Where did you get the idea that [others are critical, watching my health is important, illness is horrible, mistakes are unacceptable, it's critical to look after other people, be responsible, etc.]?" This can provide valuable opportunities to help the person understand and make sense of the good reasons behind chronic beliefs and behavior patterns. It is also very useful in helping the client to cultivate a less pejorative understanding of his or her stuckness (resistance to change). For example: "You're only doing what you learned to do." Or "Being this way was critical to being safe or getting much-needed affection and support from others." Or "So, naturally, you would think that that's the way the world works—the way other people are now." Or "So, your mother was always very critical and demanding, you couldn't do anything right. I would think that it makes great sense in that context to work incredibly hard to please everyone 24/7 so you can avoid being hurt and be spared the enormous pain that comes with criticism." Or "So, you naturally learned that others are critical. It makes sense that you would resist putting yourself out there even today, because you are just liable to get hurt again."

THERAPIST: The last thing you would want is to be oblivious to what might happen and then be caught off-guard. [amplified reflection; resonating with the identified function of health vigilance]

CLIENT: Absolutely. At least if I'm checking and watching, then I can control it. (*pause*) Well, that's kind of silly, isn't it?

THERAPIST: Say more. [Part of the client seems to be spontaneously challenging the advantage she has identified; thus, the therapist seeks to have her elaborate this potential change voice; but the therapist is waiting to hear whether the client elaborates the change position or goes back to the status quo position—in order to move flexibly with the client.]

CLIENT: Well, I know that I can't really control whether or not I get cancer. But I *know* that (*exasperated tone of voice*), and I know how silly it is to try to "catch it," but I can't stop myself from doing it. [Here, after briefly elaborating the change voice, the client quickly goes back to the status quo position, i.e., resists change; thus, the therapist must respond to what is most alive, i.e., resistance to change.]

THERAPIST: So, there's a part of you that recognizes somehow that this is a futile effort, but you feel like you have to keep trying. What is that about? Why is that so important? [double-sided reflection capturing both parts of what the client said but ending with resistance to change; and the therapist invites the client to further elaborate the good reasons behind health vigilance]

CLIENT: It would be so awful to imagine myself getting sick. My children need me. I can't be sick.

THERAPIST: . . . or die. [amplified reflection further illustrating that the therapist is tracking and with the client in what they are attempting to express in that moment]

CLIENT: Yes, I think they would be devastated and never recover from it. You can't recover from losing a mother. It changes you permanently.

THERAPIST: So, by doing everything you can to prevent this, you're caring for your children, making sure they don't suffer a terrible loss . . . You're being a great mother. [reframing health vigilance as a positive characteristic of the client; motivated by very positive intentions and values, i.e., to be a great mother]

CLIENT: But it's so silly. I feel like an idiot half the time when I'm checking my body and worrying, because I know that I imagine problems that aren't there. [Here the change position reemerges; the therapist could either seek to have the client further elaborate this or could further reflect and elaborate the status quo position.]

THERAPIST: It might sound silly from that point of view, but from another perspective it doesn't sound silly at all. You're trying to protect your kids. You're trying to spare them from suffering. What a wonderful goal, especially if you believe that this would be a devastating permanent scar. [The therapist elects to further reframe the status quo position, given the client's pejorative and self-critical construal of herself as "an idiot" i.e., attempting to help the client develop greater self-compassion and self-under-standing.]

CLIENT: Yes, I feel like it's my responsibility somehow, and that makes it hard to let go of it.

THERAPIST: So, there's a part of you that is kind of protesting a bit . . . that regards all this checking as maybe not being very useful in the end. And another very powerful part of you that is desperate to do all you can to protect your kids even if it doesn't make sense . . . because that's your job—and a very important one, at that. [summary; double-sided reflection capturing both parts of the client's dilemma]

EXPLORING GOOD THINGS ABOUT AGORAPHOBIC AVOIDANCE

THERAPIST: It may sound like a strange question, but what are some of the good things about avoiding, about not traveling, about thinking about death and worrying? [The therapist invites the client to elaborate on the positive value of the problem.]

CLIENT: (*pause*) Well, I guess if I stay at home I always have everything I need, you know.

THERAPIST: It sounds like staying at home . . . it's sort of like a sense of control over the situation. Would that fit? [The client tentatively offers one possible reason for the status quo; the therapist wants to show the client that it is safe to elaborate, so he or she reframes the statement as the client's gaining a positive sense of control.]

CLIENT: Yeah. I don't see myself as wanting to control everything but . . . or wanting to be in charge or the boss or anything like that . . . but it is kind of a control thing. I think that by staying at home I can control that no one is going to get sick . . . no one is going to die.

THERAPIST: So, it's not necessarily being a control freak. You want to control that other people aren't hurt . . . that you don't lose somebody important to you. And everybody wants control whether they say it or not. We all want to feel like we have some control over things—especially things that are dear to us. (Here the therapist is demonstrating that he or she has heard the totality of the client's expression, i.e., including the client's reluctance to use the word *control*; and the therapist then works hard to reframe and normalize this need for control.)

And later in the exploration.

THERAPIST: And another thing I think I hear is that when you do think about going somewhere else or doing something spontaneous . . . there's this chain of worries . . . "Well, what if this . . . ?" or "Where's the hospital?" These thoughts start to race. Is that right? [Here the therapist is making a suggestion, based on the conversation, about other possible bad things about change in order to further the client's exploration of the status quo, i.e., staying at home, in this case.]

CLIENT: Yeah, so I guess I don't have to worry . . . I don't have to worry about things in general.

THERAPIST: A good thing about not traveling and staying close to home is that you don't have to worry. (*The client laughs.*) And what's it like to worry like that? [The therapist is coming alongside the client's legitimate and understandable need to protect herself by staying close to home; and then inviting her to elaborate further.]

CLIENT: It's exhausting . . . It's mentally, emotionally, and physically exhausting to be thinking all those things all the time. I go away, I can't sleep, I worry about things, I get all upset, I'm not myself, I worry that people will look and go, "Oh, what's wrong with her?" (*sarcastically*)

THERAPIST: So, staying close to home allows you to worry less, sleep better . . . physically you feel better. (*pause*) And it's draining. So, you prevent yourself from feeling emotionally and physically drained. [Here the therapist is emphasizing the merits of the status quo position in order to help the client both feel free and safe to explore these further and to help the client develop a more compassionate and understanding view of her resistance to change; the reflection also has a quality of validation, i.e., "No wonder you are doing what you are doing."]

CLIENT: And I feel . . . there's that old confident me. At home, I've got everything at my disposal. I'm in control. You know. So, this is me. And when I'm away . . . When I'm at home it's like I'm the mom. And when I'm away it's like I'm the little girl that wants my mom. [The client elaborates further and provides a powerful metaphor to illustrate the allure of staying at home, i.e., resisting change.]

THERAPIST: (*softly*) You feel really helpless when you're away from home. [amplified reflection capturing what is most alive in the client's statement]

CLIENT: (*softly*) Yeah, that's a good way of describing it.

THERAPIST: So, by not going away, it protects you from feeling helpless

. . . from feeling like you're the little girl. [Again, this statement shows the therapist tracking and validating the powerful needs that are being met by the client's reluctance to travel away from home; again, it has a sense-making quality of "no wonder" or "of course."]

When the therapist reframes problematic views and reactions in this way, it also reduces the client's pejorative perceptions of resistance to change and communicates a positive view of these experiences. Clients often hold pejorative perceptions of ambivalence and resistance to change. They frequently express frustration with themselves, or become overtly self-critical, at continuing to think/act in ways that they are painfully and acutely aware are self-defeating ("I know this is ridiculous/wrong/doesn't make sense, but I do it anyway. How crazy is that?"). Therefore, the therapist holding and reflecting a more com-

> *Having a compassionate and accepting view of resistance to change counters the client's pejorative self-views.*

passionate and accepting view of resistance to change as understandable, normal, and informative can be a powerful antidote to the client's pejorative, self-critical attitudes to the persistence of self-defeating behavior.

In fact, therapist compassion and positive reframing of symptoms or problematic patterns often translate into more positive client self-perceptions and internalization of greater self-compassion. For example, a young woman with social anxiety who was initially highly self-critical about being anxious, after several sessions of working to understand and reframe these reactions, reported, "Now there is a space right after my anxiety is triggered and before what happens next. And in that space I remind myself that there's a reason—that the anxiety is just trying to help me to avoid being embarrassed. It's trying to protect me. Before, I used to think I was just crazy, abnormal, and stupid to do this to myself." Holding this more compassionate attitude may also be a very distinct, unexpected, and unique experience both for clients whose history has been marked by the absence of such responses from others and for those who typically encounter helpers who are primarily (or exclusively) interested in hearing only from the part of them that desires change. And unexpected experiences have stronger affective consequences and are more likely to be deeply processed than expected ones (Westra, Aviram, Barnes, & Angus, 2010).

Finally, in exploring and understanding the motives underlying the problem, it is also not unusual for clients to bring in developmental experiences that shaped the assumptions and behavioral patterns expressed in the problem. Understanding these can lead the client to further "make sense" of a problem that often seems nonsensical to him or her and renders the problematic response, assumptions, or pattern understandable, adaptive, and necessary in view of his or her experiences. This can often be experienced as soothing and validating for clients and can free them to explore their own beliefs and choices. For example, in the illustration above of the client beset with worry, the client noted that her mother was highly dominating, critical, demanding, and guilt-inducing. Bringing this into the exploration of the functions of her worry served to make sense of her chronic feelings of elevated responsibility and the subordination of her own needs to the service of others, with worry and vigilance to others' needs as an important vehicle for fulfilling the expectations of others, thereby ensuring and maintaining important connections with them.

Finally, another client with severe isolation and depression, when prompted with "What are the good things about keeping to yourself?," stated, "It keeps me from getting hurt." She then described a lifelong pattern beginning in childhood of moving around a lot and losing friends to whom she had become attached. She related that this left her feeling very hurt and reluctant to make new friends, feelings that her parents minimized and failed to recognize, soothe, or validate. The therapist helped the client validate the adaptive nature of isolation, in that "it protects you from having to go through the pain and risk of getting close to others just to end up losing them."

The Multifaceted Nature of Empathy

Thus, the process of engaging with the exploration (i.e., the empathic listening, validation, and embodying of the core facilitative conditions outlined by Rogers, 1975) is as important as the outcome of that exploration. A great deal is being communicated in the *process* of empathic reflection and validation, including:

- "I understand."
- "I want to know you."
- "Your thoughts and feelings are important and can be trusted."
- "It is safe."
- "I regard you highly."
- "I care for and about you."
- "Your beliefs, feelings, and actions are understandable."
- "It's okay to express difficult feelings or things you don't like about yourself."
- "I trust you to come up with your own answers."
- "You can do it."
- "You are the expert on your experience."

- "Only you can know."
- "I accept you and will not judge you even if you come up with something you typically find unacceptable to others or to yourself."

In other words, empathy is complex and multifaceted and can serve many functions that go well beyond maintaining a positive working alliance (Angus & Kagan, 2009; Watson, Goldman, & Vanaerschot, 1998). For instance, empathic responding facilitates clients' self-reflection in therapy and acknowledges that they can know themselves, evaluate their beliefs and behaviors, and make choices about change and how best to enhance the quality of their lives (Rogers, 1975; Taylor, 1990). That is, empathy unleashes the clients' potential to heal themselves (see Chapter 11 for further elaboration on the functions and use of empathic reflection). In the case of empathic reflection to better understand resistance to change, with greater self-understanding and affirmation of the positive motives underlying seemingly negative behaviors or ways of being, clients can then more freely make decisions about how well the behavior is working to meet these vital needs. They can then contemplate whether there are other ways of meeting these core needs that are less self-destructive. Such alternatives frequently emerge when the client more fully understands and appreciates the value of his or her resistance to change.

Empathy is communicated through both verbal and nonverbal behaviors, and the two should be congruent. Incongruence, such as saying the right thing but not meaning it, is easily detected by the client, who typically responds to the underlying or intended message. That is, one's words and underlying intention can be discordant, resulting in communicating a mixed message to the client. For example, the therapist might say "You get to decide" but be covertly really hoping or wanting to ensure that the decision inclines toward change. In MI parlance, this is referred to as "words without music" (Rollnick & Miller, 1995).

Conversely, it is also possible to have music without (or with only a few) words. One highly effective CBT therapist I supervised would be quite silent in the presence of client resistance, often remaining silent for several minutes (which felt like an eternity when observing the session). After this and when the client finished expressing his or her concerns about change or treatment, the therapist would come out with a highly accurate and supportively delivered summary that captured the essence of the client's concern. Raters of the tapes for therapist empathy would repeatedly be quite surprised at the therapist's summary and would remark ('Oh, she was listening after all'). In supervision, when I would replay such instances and ask the therapist what he or she was hearing and thinking during those times (with the goal of helping the therapist verbally express empathy during these times), I too was quite surprised to realize that he or she was very clearly listening and highly attentive to what the client was attempting to communicate. I suspect that despite his or her silence, the therapist may nonetheless have been communicating receptivity and attentiveness to the client nonverbally and then confirming this to the client through an accurate summary.

While I am not advocating silence in response to client expressions of concern about change, the main point here is that the intention of being receptive and open to hearing clients' concerns seems to be relatively more important than using the right words. In other words, cultivating the spirit underlying MI is more important than learning the mechanics, that is, particular questions or responses. The techniques and suggestions (e.g., questions to evoke change talk, questions to explore ambivalence) are ways of cultivating or accessing an underlying mindset, attitude, or way of being that reflects client-centeredness and the MI spirit.

RESISTANCE TO CHANGE IN DEPRESSION

Similar methods can be used for understanding the perpetuation of depression. The following is an excerpt from MI work with a young man who presented with recurrent major depressive episodes and who had not responded to a previous course of counseling. This client suffered his most recent episode of depression after his girlfriend of 3 years had moved overseas for work while the client remained in Canada. He also had a history of being bullied repeatedly in elementary school. He complained that his life always seems to be filled with chaos—chaotic eating, sleeping, school attendance, etc. And he reported feeling "I have no control." Again, the dialogue is annotated to reflect how the therapist hears and responds from the perspective of working with ambivalence.

> THERAPIST: So, there's a lot of chaos around you right now. This might sound like a strange question but I'm wondering what, if anything, is 'good' about chaos? [The therapist is working to elicit good things about resistance to change.]
>
> CLIENT: I feel like, in a weird way, I create chaos.
>
> THERAPIST: So, there's a part of you that needs things to be chaotic because . . . [encouraging elaboration to keep the exploration moving]
>
> CLIENT: I'm afraid of success. It's not so much that things have gone badly for me when I have managed to get things together, but people don't support me as much when I'm doing well.
>
> THERAPIST: So, when things are out of control, people help you more

. . . support you more. Creating chaos is a way of connecting with others . . . showing them that you need and want them around. [The therapist is reframing "chaos creation" as an important way of meeting a basic need for feeling connected to others.]

CLIENT: My family doesn't really show affection . . . They don't really show that they care a lot—except when I'm in trouble.

THERAPIST: And you want to be close to them. You want and need them to show they care—all the time, not just when you're in trouble. [The therapist again reinforces the value of the need for connection, which further encourages the client to elaborate.]

CLIENT: Like, my mom was great when I was bullied in school. She was really in my corner, really proactive, and fought like a pit bull to protect me and do her best to make sure it stopped.

THERAPIST: So, she can be a really strong ally, and you miss that. You only see that side of her when it's clear that you're struggling. (*pause*) And you can't ask for what you need without showing that you're struggling . . . that things are chaotic. Being out of control is a way of getting support without having to ask for it. [The therapist is guessing at a key function of the "creating chaos" behavior, namely, receiving support without having to risk asking for support; but the attitude is one where the client is free to dismiss this guess or elaborate on it.]

CLIENT: I feel bad asking.

THERAPIST: Say more about that. [The therapist sees that the client does seem to resonate with the guess about one possible function of "creating chaos" and therefore asks him to elaborate.]

CLIENT: It's weak . . . needy. I don't deserve it, and it's weak to need it. Like, I don't ask my mom to come over and help me with the apartment—even though that would be really helpful, given that I haven't been able to do anything lately.

THERAPIST: It makes a lot of sense that you aren't comfortable expressing what you need from your mom directly. Even though there's a part of you that wants and needs support and knows from past experience how to get it, the larger part of you says "I'm not good enough to deserve it." [summary reflection indicating that the therapist is tracking all parts of the client's ambivalence; also an attempt at validation of another identified issue, namely, not asking directly for support]

And in a subsequent discussion of his chaotic sleep patterns, in particular, the client reported feeling very frustrated with himself for staying awake until 3 or 4 in the morning and then sleeping in and napping later in the day. Initially, we explored education on sleep hygiene, which he reported finding useful but failed to implement. He was also able to articulate the many downsides to his erratic sleep patterns, including missing classes, being constantly exhausted, disrupted eating habits, perpetuation of his depressed mood, and so on. That is, despite recognizing and presenting this as a problem to be solved, he was reluctant to take steps to change it. Thus, here the focus of our work on ambivalence centered on a specific aspect of his depression—sleep habits.

THERAPIST: What helps about staying up late?

CLIENT: I feel so much more productive at night. I have a lot of energy then.

THERAPIST: And this is probably something that is most welcome, given your general lack of energy or feeling productive since being depressed. [validation, i.e., "it's understandable"; also a reframing, i.e., on the surface this seems like a problem—and it is to some extent—but there are elements of it that are also a solution]

CLIENT: Yes. And it's quiet at night. Like, my parents are great, but they talk a lot. When they're awake, they're talking.

THERAPIST: And you need some peace and quiet sometimes. Some time to yourself—a break from the noise. And you can get this at night when they're asleep and during the day when you're asleep. [The therapist demonstrates that she has heard the client's identified functions of not sleeping at night and this encourages the client to further elaborate.]

CLIENT: Yes. It feels good to sleep in, too. I feel indulgent.

THERAPIST: So, it's kind of a "treat" in a way. A way of spoiling yourself . . . being kind to yourself . . . giving yourself something that feels good. That makes a lot of sense, especially when you've been feeling so rotten. [more validation, more reframing, i.e., uncovering and resonating with the positive value of the seemingly negative behavior/pattern]

CLIENT: And then I don't have to think about how I'm feeling, either.

THERAPIST: So, a kind of anesthetic . . . a break from the pain. So, even though you're tired during the day and may not be as productive as you could be, it's worth it in a way for some quiet time . . . some time to yourself . . . a much-needed break. [further demonstration that the therapist can hear the functions of the "negative" behavior; here the therapist also pulls the two sides of the ambivalence together—develops discrepancy—to help the client reflect on the value of the behavior in the context of the costs of the behavior; this is not done to "show the client that it's not worth it" but rather to further the client's own exploration of his ambivalence.]

CLIENT: Actually, no.

THERAPIST: You don't agree that it's worth it.

CLIENT: It erodes my ability to study because I'm so exhausted all the time and I really need to make good grades. And I can't just bury my head in the ground and pretend that nothing is wrong, no matter how good it feels. [Here, the client rejects the therapist's guess, but the discrepancy prompts him to further consider his position of the value of the status quo; the therapist then responds by acknowledging the emergence of the change position and encouraging its elaboration; the therapist would, however, be prepared to move flexibly with the client, were resistance to change to reemerge.]

In this case, a consistent effort to understand, reframe, and validate the problem led to the client's beginning to express the other side of his ambivalence, that is, change talk. He then began to brainstorm about how to change his sleep habits. Moreover, recognizing his unconventional sleep habits as a way of being good to himself, the client then began to brainstorm other, less problematic, ways of self-soothing (playing with his cat, going out with friends, etc.). One can also use the previously identified good things or functions of the problem to help strengthen self-efficacy and bolster resolve in approaching change when the client shifts to more active consideration of change. For example, "What about that part of you that says,' You need this, you deserve this, it's going to feel good!' What do you say to that?" That is, on hearing good things, you can more effectively combat obstacles that arise when the client sets out to make change (this is further discussed in Chapter 8).

In my experience, there are often important needs being met and important messages being communicated by the behaviors characterizing depression. For example, withdrawal can be an effort to reduce unrelenting demands and expectations of others, to reduce aversive stimuli or to take much-needed respite. Consider, for example, a client with severe depression and hopelessness whom a therapist consulted with me about since he was highly resistant to treatment—refusing to be involved in any therapy offerings from their CBT treatment program and essentially unwilling to help himself in any way. This was very concerning to program staff in view of the severity of his depression. The therapist explained that this middle-aged man had had a major accident that left him so permanently disabled that he was unable to return to his former employment and successful career as a lawyer. He was the father of a young child and the sole income earner in his household. I asked the therapist, "What might the depression be trying to say?" The therapist thought for a while and then, with a severe expression and forceful tone of voice, turned to me and said, "Leave me alone! Back off!," to which I replied: "I see. Stop all your nattering about how I could look on the bright side and 'there's hope for the future.' I feel miserable. I've lost everything. I need time! Don't you get that?"

This led to a very productive discussion about how to hear this potential message and respond. As we considered this fellow's situation, we both felt tearful at the prospect of putting ourselves in his place. We shuddered to think about the astounding implications of the accident for the client's sense of self, role, feelings of efficacy, and the future. We decided that the best thing the therapist might offer this client was the most difficult thing of all—to have the courage to be with and bear witness to this man's enormous suffering; to help him give voice to his agony, fears, and concerns and provide critical space to help him begin to make sense out of this tragedy and to sort out the meanings and implications for him and his future (free from any demands for him to be different or change). The therapist decided to see the man for individual therapy sessions with this intention and happily reported that she "couldn't shut him up." The client apparently appeared visibly relieved and remarked that he had no other place to talk in this way since he felt a need to be strong and brave and not burden his family with his troubled feelings. Understood from his perspective, it was not the case that this gentleman did not wish to engage in therapy; rather, he had no desire (very understandably) to engage with a treatment that began with an assumption and expectation that he should change and did not make room for his important need to resist change. Only when an effort was made to understand and hear the good reasons for not changing did that pave the way for his more active engagement in treatment.

In other instances, depression can be a means of attempting to elicit support from others, preserve relationships, and keep others close. Consider the case of a woman with a long history of experiencing neglect in close relationships that was particularly acute (and ongoing) in her highly enmeshed relationship with her mother. A major aspect of her self-definition was the need to be highly successful, and she felt very frightened that others could not accept her if she did not succeed.

She made substantial progress in understanding the impact of these experiences in contributing to her longstanding problems with anxiety and depression, and in fact she had recently reconnected with her father. Her mother had been separated from her father years earlier, was highly critical of him, and effectively prevented my client from having any significant relationship with him. After significant progress in reducing her self-criticism, improving her self-care, reconnecting with her father (who was surprisingly experienced as caring and compassionate by the client), and achieving some healthier boundaries in her relationship with her mother, my client experienced a major relapse in her depression. This was indeed puzzling to her, and we explored together its possible meaning (good things).

CLIENT: One thing I've noticed is that I typically don't reach out when I'm feeling troubled. I keep things like that to myself. I have always felt like I have to be the strong one. But now I have been calling up my family a lot and talking about my feelings.

THERAPIST: So, that's different. You're kind of experimenting with something new here.

CLIENT: Yes.

THERAPIST: And what have you discovered?

CLIENT: (*tearfully*) That they are there for me. Everyone has been so supportive and kind. And they don't seem to care about what I do. I even asked them what they would think of me if I quit my job because I really don't like it, and they said that they would be there for me—they would support me in whatever I decided.

THERAPIST: Aha! Maybe they really do care about you beyond your abilities. Maybe you don't have to be highly successful in order to be loved.

CLIENT: Exactly. I always felt like I was the magnet holding everything together in my family. Everyone was so focused on me and my success, my achievements—so proud of me.

THERAPIST: What pressure! And so to realize that you may not have to play that role any more is shocking in many ways.

CLIENT: Yes. I almost don't know what to do with it.

THERAPIST: I don't know if this fits at all, but maybe by being "sick" and "in need" it sounds like you got some answers to a vitally important question. You've been doing so much work on expanding who you are and who you want to be beyond this narrow suffocating self-definition as a doctor. And talk is cheap—anyone can say they will be there for you—but by actually being in need and reaching out, you really have a chance to find out if other people will be there for you, regardless of whether or not you are a "success."

CLIENT: That makes a lot of sense, because the one person I didn't call was my partner [who lived in a different province].

THERAPIST: Because you are confident in her response.

CLIENT: Exactly. I have no doubt about her and that she accepts me, no matter what. And I also called my former mentor. She was always so "proud" of me and praising me for my giftedness.

THERAPIST: So, if you did quit, didn't do what she wanted for you, would that be okay with her—if you're not this person she groomed you to be? Can you really be free to make your own choices?

Thus, as these examples illustrate, symptoms can have meanings and serve as important communication devices. Understandably, then, efforts to take these away can be met with resistance until the meaning of them is understood and recognized. In such situations, it can be far more effective to reframe seemingly negative, maladaptive behavior as an adaptive effort driven by positive intentions and as containing an important message to be explored and heard before change can be considered.

THERAPIST FEARS OF EXPLORING THE STATUS QUO

Therapists learning MI can sometimes articulate anxiety about reflecting, encouraging, or siding with the reasons for not changing. This can indeed feel like an unfamiliar position, particularly for therapists who are used to being more directive and are highly adept at and more familiar with advocating for change. There can be a fear that supporting the client's understanding of the good reasons for not changing might facilitate his or her decision not to change or be giving the client "permission" to not change.

First, it is important to remember that decisions about changing one's behavior can only rest with the client. Assuming that therapists can give clients permission is falsely assuming that one can usurp the client's role as the authority on whether to change. Moreover, in exploring the advantages to the status quo, therapists are not in fact "reinforcing" maladaptive behavior (e.g., avoidance, isolation, drinking) but rather accepting and validating the motivations underlying the behavior. One can support the client's inherent desire for safety and connection with others, for example, while facilitating the client in his or her own determination of whether the current means of accomplishing these ends are sufficient, useful, a fit with his or her values, or the like.

> *In exploring the advantages of the status quo, therapists are not in fact "reinforcing" or "agreeing with" clients' maladaptive behavior.*

There are also times in using MI when the client decides that change is not a good idea and is not preferred over the status quo. However, these times are relatively rare in my experience since people are inherently motivated to attain positive things in their lives (Rogers, 1965). And when people do decide not to change, this is also consistent with the client's self-determination, that is, the client gets to decide not to change or that changing does not make sense.

It may also be tempting to view MI methods as a clever way of overcoming resistance to change so that one can move more productively to helping the client take action to achieve change. While this is of course ultimately true, it can represent a subtle but very important deviation from MI spirit. Any therapist agenda for change, no matter how well intentioned, can interfere with communicating and embodying the sincerity, genuineness, and congruence that underlie the spirit of MI. For example, I recall working with a therapist practicing CBT in the context of a controlled research trial (comparing CBT with and without MI) who wanted to do a cost–benefit analysis with his client. I was of course very reluctant to have him use this technique for a client who was not supposed to receive MI in this study—until I had him describe his intentions and goals in using this technique. The therapist indicated that the client had a number of mistaken positive beliefs about worry. He hoped that working through these with a cost–benefit analysis would help her see these misleading assumptions more clearly, thereby allowing her to challenge these misperceptions. I told him to go ahead since the crucial MI spirit was missing and therefore this could not be considered MI.

SUMMARY

Effectively managing resistance to change can be a very difficult skill to cultivate since resistance often and naturally pulls for therapist efforts to influence, control, and defeat such objections to change. In contrast, working effectively with resistance to change involves reframing it as containing important information to be understood and integrated. Resistance to change reflects positive motivations—clients' efforts to meet vital and universal needs and to do the best they can with what they have learned. In itself, this can be therapeutic for clients who are often frustrated and confused by their own (seemingly nonsensical) resistance to change. It enables clients to accept and approach their objections to change and to cultivate a more compassionate view of themselves, their existing ways of being, and their efforts to change.

Moreover, when resistance to change is approached with this more accepting and understanding attitude, it is not at all uncommon for change talk (arguments for change, objections to the status quo) to emerge spontaneously. As individuals more fully understand the reasons for and motives underlying the persistence of the problem they are seeking to change, they are better equipped to critically examine and question the adequacy and sufficiency of these ("old") approaches in meeting their goals. They can begin the process of deciding whether existing beliefs and chronic behavior patterns continue to serve them in the present or whether more effective and satisfying approaches are possible and could be developed. And having the client (rather than the therapist) develop and make the arguments for change is a very important process to nurture in increasing motivation for change. Evoking and then consolidating such change talk represent the focus of the next chapter.

7

❦

Evoking and Elaborating
Change Talk

As we have seen in the preceding chapter, rolling with resistance to change often elicits active contemplation of the part of the person that desires change. That is, the part of the person desiring and arguing for change seems to emerge and becomes more alive. In this process, the person often begins to contemplate and get in touch with his or her core values, authentic and desired identity, and valued life directions. In essence, clients begin to explore "who they really are" and "what they genuinely and sincerely want." These questions can often feel novel and foreign to clients continually caught up in and distracted by chronic and automatic patterns of anxious responding. Anxiety is a dominant response system in the brain and hijacks other less critical pursuits that are not central to survival (such as one's values, desires, and preferences). Thus, continually responding to emergencies and striving for security naturally precludes such critical self-examination. In MI, the therapist plays an important role in evoking and supporting the contemplation of such questions about what the client authentically values, desires, and wishes to strive for (reasons for change) and how the problem is an obstacle to pursuing such valued directions and constructing a more satisfying life (i.e., the downsides of the status quo).

Thus, the overarching goal at this stage is to help clients focus on articulating and elaborating change talk (reasons to change, downsides to the status quo) and to help them more fully understand and embrace valued directions for change. Regardless of whether change talk occurs spontaneously or is elicited by the therapist, therapists should seek to elaborate and strengthen it. Initially, such change talk can feel very weak and fragile and requires strengthening through invitations (reflections and questions) to elaborate. Such strengthening helps clients to build resolve for change by bringing important motives for change into awareness and enables them to engage more fully with these incentives. Increased awareness of these authentic motivations for change is also a critical resource that encourages clients to exert greater resistance to returning to the status quo position when they begin to change.

EXPLORING AND ELABORATING THE COSTS OF STAYING THE SAME AND THE BENEFITS OF CHANGE

One of the distinctive features of MI that differentiates it from client-centered counseling is the focus on eliciting and elaborating of change talk (i.e., speech that reflects the client's desires, abilities, reasons, needs, and commitments to change; Amrhein et al., 2003). Here, the therapist evokes (or encourages spontaneously emerging) change talk and elaborates it through empathic reflection. The prompts on working with ambivalence shown in Table 5.1 (on the right-hand side) can serve as useful points of inquiry and or elaboration of change talk. Further possible points of entry into this dialogue that are recommended by Miller and Rollnick (2002) are reproduced in Table 7.1. This list has been adapted for work with individuals with anxiety and depression.

Again, it is the elaboration of change talk and the awareness of authentic desired directions that is important in MI. In other words, the goal is not to have a superficial laundry list of downsides to the status quo or advantages to change. Accordingly, the overall spirit of curiosity and exploration in the service of facilitating client awareness and decision making is more important than the particular questions or prompts used. Therapists should also avoid the "question-and-answer trap" (Miller & Rollnick, 2002), since this can create an atmosphere of inquisition and information gathering, with the therapist in the role as expert. This can detract from creating a self-reflective atmosphere of client exploration of reasons for change.

Stated differently, enhancing motivation is not the product of some type of straightforward, linear, or mathematical logic (e.g., "There are 10 pros to change and 5 cons to change—therefore I'm going to change"). Increasing resolve for change is not about quantifying or listing downsides but rather has much more to do with the client experiencing and becoming more fully aware of the costs of the problem and envisioning how life would be without it. As such, emotional engagement with the identified advantages of change and problems with not changing is crucial. Thus, questions and prompts for elaborating the change position should be considered possible springboards for beginning the critical process of such engagement; but they

TABLE 7.1. Open Questions to Evoke Change Talk

Disadvantages of the status quo
- "What worries you about your current situation?"
- "What makes you think that you need to something about your anxiety/ depression?"
- "What difficulties or hassles have you had in relation to your anxiety/ depression?"
- "What is there about your anxiety/depression that you or other people might see as reasons for concern?"
- "In what ways does this concern you?"
- "How has this stopped you from doing what you want to do in life?"
- "What do you think will happen if you don't change anything?"

Advantages of change
- "How would you like for things to be different?"
- "What would be the good things about being less anxious/depressed?"
- "What would you like your life to be like 5 years from now?"
- "If you could make this change immediately, by magic, how might things be better for you?"
- "The fact that you're here indicates that at least part of you thinks it's time to do something. What are the main reasons you see for making a change?"
- "What would be the advantages of making this change?"

Optimism about change
- "What makes you think that, if you did decide to make a change, you could do it?"
- "What encourages you that you can change if you want to?"
- "What do you think would work for you, if you decided to change?"
- "When else in your life have you made a significant change like this? How did you do it?"
- "How confident are you that you can make this change?"
- "What personal strengths do you have that will help you succeed?"
- "Who could offer you helpful support in making this change?"

Intention to change
- "I can see that you're feeling stuck at the moment. What's going to have to change?"
- "What do you think you might do?"
- "How important is this to you? How much do you want to do this?"
- "What would you be willing to try?"
- "Of the options I've mentioned, which one sounds like it fits you best?"
- "Never mind the 'how' for right now—what do you want to have happen?"
- "So, what do you intend to do?"

Note. Adapted from Miller and Rollnick (2002, p. 79). Copyright 2002 by The Guilford Press. Adapted by permission.

are not the process itself. Rather, the goal of building resolve for change is primarily achieved through curious and patient elaboration and close, careful empathic listening. Catching the implied meanings and the unspoken feelings associated with the costs of the problem (and what it would be and feel like to be one's true self/ without the problem) is critical fod-

Increasing resolve for change is not about quantifying downsides but rather making the client more fully aware of the costs of the problem and envisioning how life would be without it.

der for promoting further client exploration and helping clients get into experiential contact with these concerns/desires.

It is also important to seek to identify downsides to the problem and benefits to change that are significant from the client's perspective rather than the therapist's point of view or values. The therapist can add suggestions of possible downsides for the client's consideration (and make guesses about others that are implied in the client's statements), but only downsides to the problem or advantages to change that resonate with the client should be elaborated. I recall supervising a therapist using MI who was herself a young mother. She could not believe that her client, a mother with young children, did not identify the impact of her severe agoraphobic avoidance on her children as a potential problem and did not resonate with this when the therapist inquired about it. The therapist had to work to bracket her own values in the service of being more curious about benefits to change that did have meaning for this particular client and the downsides to anxiety that the client identified with and felt more deeply.

RESPONDING TO CHANGE TALK

Table 7.2 contains a summary of the suggestions offered by Miller and Rollnick (2002) for responding to change talk in order to invite the client to further elaborate on it, thereby strengthening it. I have adapted this list of questions for work with anxiety concerns and have supplemented it with other suggestions that may also be useful.

As noted previously, while many individuals identify a range of costs to anxiety/depression and the benefits of changing, not all of these have personal meaning or significance. Emotional intensity and the way a downside is expressed can provide information on its potential significance to the client (e.g., tearfulness, becoming sullen or quiet, anger, squirming). In general, the therapist should try to illuminate and grasp the emotional significance of the problem (and the advantages to changing it) since emo-

TABLE 7.2. Responding to Change Talk

Asking for elaboration

- "Say more about that—In what ways is this a problem? How often does it occur? How significant are the problems that the anxiety creates?)"
- "Can you give me a specific example of what you mean? When was the last time this occurred? What happened? What did you notice? How did it feel?"
- "What goes on inside when you consider living with this?"
- "What is it like to be this way?"
- " [If the client indicates the presence of emotion, e.g., sighing, tearful] "Heavy sigh—what is that about? Talk from the tears?"
- "What exactly don't you like about . . . ?"
- "What else . . . ?"
- "I see how it makes some sense to stay the same. Is there any price that you pay for that?"
- "Are there any holes in the argument for not changing, or does it make 100% sense?"
- "You mentioned that worry helps you to feel in control. How well does it accomplish that important goal? 10% helpful? 100% helpful?" Or "You mentioned that being depressed is a way of getting support and connecting to others. How successful is it at meeting that need?"

Querying extremes

- "Suppose you continue on as you have been, without changing. What do you imagine are the worst things that might happen?"
- "What might be the best results you could imagine if you make a change?"

Looking back

- "What were things like for you before you became depressed/anxious? What were you like back then?"
- "What are the differences between the Pat [the client's name] of 10 years ago and the Pat of today?"
- "How has your anxiety/depression changed you as a person . . . stopped you from growing . . . from moving forward?"

Looking forward under conditions of change and no change

- "If the future persisted exactly as it is now, what would be bad about that for you?"
- "Is there a time in the future when being as you are now just wouldn't do for you anymore . . . the price would be too high? [If yes:] Describe."
- "If the anxiety/depression was no longer a problem, what would be good about that?"

Exploring goals and values

- "What's distressing about being this way?"
- "In what ways is it not okay to see yourself/be this way?"

(continued)

TABLE 7.2. (*continued*)

- "In what ways exactly does this hurt you? . . . walk me through that."
- "Is this something trivial, or is it more important than that?"
- "How important, on a scale of 1 to 10, is [this cost of not changing/benefit of change]? Why an X and not a Y [lower score]?" [e.g., "Why a 7 and not a 2?"]
- "To what degree does being this way fit or not fit with what you really want in life . . . with where you are going . . . who you really are or what you value?"
- "If you were to dream or fantasize for a moment about what life could be like that's different from the way things are now, what picture would you paint? Why are those things important to you?"
- "Is there anything you want that you aren't getting by staying the same? Describe in detail what those things are. What are you after?"
- "Of the costs to your anxiety, what are the most troubling ones for you? Which are the most painful?"
- "Speak from the part of you that is really pained/distressed/suffering/hurt by this."

Note. Based on Miller and Rollnick (2002).

tionally laden and personally significant costs (i.e., ones that "touch" or "move" the person) are much more important to elaborate than more intellectualized or theoretical responses. This is because emotionally laden costs to the problem and benefits of change typically impinge the greatest on the client's values. In other words, a given cost to the problem arouses distress when it impedes or interferes with the attainment of goals or aims central to the person. Emotions are significant markers of something valuable to the individual, indicating that that course of action has particular value or important meaning to him or her (e.g., Greenberg, 2002). If the presence of significant emotion is evident (e.g., sighing, tearfulness, head shaking), the therapist should notice this and ask the client to elaborate further (e.g., "Heavy sigh. What is that about?," "Can you speak from the tears?"). Or, to evoke this, the therapist can ask, "What goes on inside as you talk about this?" Relatedly, the use of strong language can also signify a meaningful consequence of the problem/benefit to change—for example, "I have *no* life," "I'm *cheating* others because of my avoidance," "I *hate* it that I'm acting fake," or "I would *love* to be able to . . . "

THE IMPORTANCE OF VALUES

Accordingly, therapists should not merely help clients articulate the costs of the problem and the benefits to change but work especially to help them consider these costs/benefits in the context of their values and valued directions. Values are very strong influences on behavior. Authentic values and valued directions can be a major impetus for considering change since we will endure and sacrifice much for our values. And the awareness of what we really want/who we really are can produce significant momentum in enduring the difficult steps that must be taken in order to change. That is, increased awareness of one's inherent values can considerably strengthen resolve for change in order to live consistently with one's vision of a meaningful, satisfying life direction. Moreover, the status quo position often pulls people in directions that are inconsistent with what they genuinely believe, value, and desire (e.g., "The anxiety has you distance myself from people, and yet you really want to connect with and be closer to others"). Thus, helping clients become more fully aware of their most heartfelt values and inherently prized life directions is an important task.

Accordingly, in exploring and elaborating the arguments for change, the therapist preferentially seeks to deepen an understanding of exactly how the problem causes distress or interferes with actualizing of the client's values. For example, if the client states that "I can't relax because I'm worried all the time" or "Cleaning all the time is time-consuming," the therapist can become curious about the significance or importance of these downsides by asking, "And how important is that? Are you thinking 'Well, relaxation/time is overrated anyway,' or is it more significant to you than that?" If it is more significant, "Why? How exactly is not being able to relax/the time-consuming element of the OCD a problem? How is it hurting you? What would be better if you could relax / didn't have to clean all the time? Talk from the part of you that is bothered by not being able to relax / all the time you spend cleaning." If the identified disadvantage(s) is not personally significant, then help the client identify other problems with the status quo or benefits to change that might be significant. For example, "What hurts you the most about being depressed? . . . about the anxiety?," "If this problem continued, what would be the biggest casualty . . . and how important would that be? . . . How difficult would that be to live with?," "What is the painful price the depression or anxiety exacts on your life?"

Highlighting clients' values can strengthen their resolve to change.

Using externalizing language can also be helpful when discussing the problem (status quo position). For example: "The anxiety tells you that . . . ," "The depression tries to convince you that . . . ," "The part of you that argues against change says . . . ," and, using internalizing language for the change position, "I really want . . . ," "I don't believe that . . . ," "I don't agree that . . . ," or "I'm more like. . . . " Using externalizing language removes the problem from the person to a certain extent, reduces his or her identification with it, and seems to facilitate greater free-dom in identifying alternative positions. Also, using internalizing language to articulate change talk facilitates identification with intrinsic values. For example, "The anxiety tells you that you can prevent rejection by avoiding people, but it seems that you might not agree. Can you say more?" or "The depression argues that it's best to not be around people when you feel this way, but part of you is doubting that. Is that right?"

Moreover, given that clients often have limited awareness of the values implicitly guiding their behavior or have often not explicitly articulated these valued life directions, it can be helpful to bring in some brief psycho-education on the importance of elaboration of the change voice to further encourage this work. This is particularly helpful with those who have trou-ble accessing their values or elaborating the significance of the downsides to the problem or with those who become self-critical at not being aware of their values or being able to access what they genuinely desire for their life. For example:

> "So, this voice sounds new and sounds like it has important things to say. It seems that this voice gets drowned out a lot of the time by the anxiety/depression, which seems to seize the microphone a lot. It can be important to make some space to listen to that part of you that wants things to be different . . . is angry about this . . . is unhappy about this . . . and so on. Does that make sense? [If yes:] If you're will-ing, can you speak more from that voice?"

In other words, because clients have been so preoccupied by respond-ing to threats, they have not had time or space to consider what they really want or who they genuinely are. Clients sometimes need encouragement and reassurance that the process of doing this can be difficult and take time. For example: "Something in you knows this is causing you pain, interfering with what you really want, or else you would not be here. It might be tough at first, but try accessing and speaking from that voice so that we can hear what it has to say—bring it into the conversation."

CLINICAL EXAMPLES

Consider the following vignette of a mother with two young children who suffered with recurrent and severe depressive episodes (requiring hospital-ization on two previous occasions). She identified numerous disadvanta-geous to overcoming her depression and made persuasive arguments for the status quo. However, powerful incentives for change were uncovered when the therapist inquired about the downsides to her depression.

THERAPIST: There's an incredibly powerful argument here for staying the same [provides summary]. I'm wondering why you are here at all? Why would you bother considering change and treatment?

CLIENT: (*on the verge of tears, speaking very softly*) because it hurts my children.

THERAPIST: That sounds important. Can you say it again? [picking up on emotional markers indicating the presence of personally significant costs and seeking to render this awareness more salient]

CLIENT: (*with slightly more volume and clear pain*) It hurts my children.

THERAPIST: And that sounds really important somehow. I can see that that really touches something. Can you say more about how that hurts? [inviting the client to elaborate]

CLIENT: (*Begins to cry.*) I love them so much . . . They're everything to me. I feel terrible that I can't do anything with them because of how bad I feel all the time . . . I can't take them to the park, spend time with them . . . I don't do anything with them.

THERAPIST: So, you really value being a great mother, and it's tremendously painful to see yourself not doing things to nurture your kids—to be the great mom that you want and need to be.

Recognizing her children and her role as a mother as highly valued to and important for her, we spent considerable time elaborating these desires and the obstacle the depression represented to living consistently with these important values. We explored what exactly bothered her, what bothered her the most, how she felt about noticing this, things she noticed in her kids that caused her concern, how they might be feeling and what they were wanting, what she feared and would feel if her depression were to continue, what she really desired and envisioned about her parenting and the future of her family and how exactly the depression was getting in the way of realizing these goals and objectives. That is, we took time to explore, elaborate, and understand this experience and the values underlying the pain the problem was causing. At the next session, the client noted that she had spent more time with her children during the preceding week, a major change for her. Recognizing this step as an indication of moving closer to the action phase (i.e., resolving ambivalence, emerging behavioral commitment to change), I shifted to facilitating her self-efficacy and increasing her growing commitment to change by becoming curious about how she managed to accomplish this, whether she thought it made sense to continue with it, what it said about her, and so on (See Chapter 9 for further discussion of developing and processing actions toward change.)

Empathic listening is the major method employed in the elaboration. In addition to the many communicative and other functions of empathy outlined earlier (and discussed further in Chapter 11), empathic responding at this stage (when the client first begins to articulate reasons for change) also serves to "fill the room with change talk"—which, in turn, serves to consolidate resolve for change and

> *Empathic reflection fills the room with change talk, increasing the client's commitment.*

pave the way to increasing commitment to change. That is, through such responding, clients hear the arguments for change repeatedly: once when they state them, again when you reflect (and deepen) them, and again when that reflection or prompt invites further client elaboration.

In addition, therapists' reflections serve an arguably more useful role in encouraging elaboration than do questions since they build on what the client has expressed and represent guesses the therapist is making about the client's experience, values, and the like. They contain an implicit invitation for the client to elaborate—to either agree, disagree, correct, or revise in a way that helps clients further clarify their meaning and understand themselves and their experience. Using reflections rather than questions also more effectively communicates that "I am working hard to understand you," since questions involve no attempt to guess at or symbolize the person's experience. In short, even though questions are easier than searching to grasp and articulate the person's experience or meaning, reflections are much more powerful in communicating empathic understanding. Moyers and colleagues recommend that therapists using MI attempt to initiate at least two to three times as many reflections as questions (Moyers, Martin, Manuel, & Miller, 2003). In fact, in training students in MI, I find it useful to suggest that trainees spend at least one session attempting to ask as *few* questions as possible. This can be a very challenging but illuminating exercise in recognizing the difficulty of good empathic listening and cultivating MI spirit.

Consider the following illustration of elaborating change talk by using a combination of reflective listening and prompts (questions) to further explore the change position:

CLIENT: I feel insecure all the time. I've felt that way my whole life.

THERAPIST: Never confident that you're good enough.

CLIENT: It used to be about my appearance; now it's about my parenting, my health, my job, everything . . .

THERAPIST: So, in part, that's why you try to be Superman. Someone that is always doing the right thing . . . someone who is there for people—someone they can count on. [linking with information from earlier work with this client]

CLIENT: I feel like I have to have a million things on the go—be the soccer coach, the respected teacher, the great father, chairman of the board, the go-to guy for everyone who needs something.

THERAPIST: Sounds exhausting!

CLIENT: Absolutely. I'm tired all the time.

THERAPIST: Not a wonder. And there's a sense that it's relentless—it's never enough. You have to make sure that others respect you— You have to keep proving over and over that you can be counted on—that you're a good guy. [guessing at an implied downside of the status quo]

CLIENT: Exactly. I never feel relaxed, you know. I'm never confident or assured that I'm okay.

THERAPIST: And that bothers you—that that insecurity just sits there waiting to rear its head again—that what you're doing doesn't fix it. And, I'm also hearing, "I'm not okay with that." Is that right? [further guessing at feeling to elaborate the change position]

CLIENT: I never feel good enough—never happy. I'm tired of chasing my tail around all the time. I've been doing that my whole life. And it's ridiculous—the lengths I'll go to. (*Gives examples.*)

THERAPIST: It's gotten way out of hand. It's okay to be responsible— that sounds like an important part of who you are—but you go way overboard. It's your whole focus. And there may be other things you want to focus on. [further guessing, to elaborate and bring in values]

CLIENT: I don't even know what I want.

THERAPIST: Why would you? It sounds like the anxiety has had you so preoccupied and distracted with what other people want. [validating] And you've had to do that to feel good about yourself. But now you're thinking, "I don't feel good about myself—certainly not as good as I should, given all the effort I'm putting in. [developing discrepancy] And that bothers me."

CLIENT: Absolutely. I don't want to sound uncaring, but I want to think about myself for a change.

THERAPIST: To me, that doesn't sound uncaring at all. It sounds balanced. [offering a more compassionate view, but the therapist is clear that this is her own viewpoint that is being offered] How important is it to you to think about changing this, with 1 being "You know what, I complain about it once in a while, but it's really not a big deal" and 10 being "It is a huge deal?" [question to evoke further change talk]

CLIENT: Eight.

THERAPIST: So, quite important. What goes into that 8? [prompt for elaboration of reasons for change]

CLIENT: I feel like I'm not in control of my life. And I'm a guy who likes control.

THERAPIST: So, this way of operating doesn't make you feel more in control, it makes you feel less in control. [summary to highlight discrepancy] What else?

CLIENT: I think I want things, and I'm not even sure what they are right now, but I'm so focused on keeping up appearances and that feels kind of hollow—makes me feel superficial, not real.

THERAPIST: You want things that are more fulfilling—more satisfying than just trying to prove that you're okay all the time. I'm also hearing that "I may want and need some space, some freedom from all this chasing, to think about what those things might be." [prompt to develop awareness of values and begin to conceptualize action to accomplish desired changes]

NURTURING CHANGE TALK

Thus far, we have considered possible ways of responding to change talk in order to elaborate it, but there are important nuances and subtleties in furthering client consideration of the change position, that have implications for whether the client will persist with such exploration or retreat from it (and move to the status quo position). In the literature on empathic listening, there is an important concept called "the leading edge" (e.g., Martin, 1999). Here, the therapist is trying to accurately capture the client's meaning and experience while not being too far behind or too far ahead of the client. Being too far behind (e.g., just restating the client's utterances) fails to move the client forward in their exploration, while being too far ahead (overstating the utterances or including meanings or experiences that are well outside of the scope of the client's awareness or intended meaning) causes the client to respond defensively. For example, if a client starts to articulate some vague feelings of dissatisfaction with his or her spouse and the therapist says, "You are really angry. Maybe this marriage isn't working," the client is then in the position of backing off from his or her original statement in the service of correcting the therapist—for example, "I wouldn't say I'm angry—it's not that serious, really." The client's exploration of these emergent feelings is essentially interrupted by the therapist. And, in general, being too far ahead is a more serious problem than being too far behind, as the latter will tend to delay or slow the client's exploration but likely will not stop it. Thus, part of the art of reflective listening is catching implied (but present—even if only dimly) meanings and expressing these back to the client in a manner that allows the client to approach them and elaborate further.

Let's consider this important skill in the context of evoking and elaborating change talk. Recall that change talk can initially be very fragile and tentative. Thus, care must be taken to gently nurture the further expression of this type of talk and create the conditions that enable the client to say more from the change position. Being too enthusiastic or emphatic about the costs of the problem or the benefits of change, or assuming that the client's meaning is obvious, can discourage the client from elaborating further. In MI terms, if, in responding to client change talk, the therapist is too far ahead of the client's meaning, this increases the probability of engendering resistance to change and leads the client to elaborate (or defend) the status quo position. Conversely, avoiding overstating the client's meaning increases the probability of further change talk. And guessing in a way that "undershoots" the intended meaning (or accurately captures it) invites the client to safely elaborate further. Thus, while good MI practice involves working to elaborate change talk when it emerges, there is a skill and an art to doing so as well as more and less effective ways of achieving this.

Table 7.3 contains examples of possible client statements favoring change among clients struggling with anxiety. Examples of therapist responses to these statements that are overstatements and thus risk engendering resistance and client counterchange talk are then offered. These are contrasted in the final column with therapist responses that are understatements or more accurate reflections of the client's meaning and therefore are more likely to encourage further client exploration of change and to elicit further change talk.

Note that the contraindicated overstated reflections in Table 7.3 are easy for clients to disagree with and in fact encourage the client to correct the overstatement (with statements favoring the status quo), while the more tentative, less emphatic, gently inviting responses are hard to disagree with. They make it safer for clients to elaborate further. Responding to change talk in a more emphatic or overstated manner can be experienced by clients as pressure to articulate, commit to, advocate for, or agree with positions

Since initial change talk can be fragile, further expression of it must be gently nurtured.

TABLE 7.3. Therapist Responses to Client Change Talk

Client initial change talk	Therapist responses that risk eliciting counterchange talk	Therapist responses that nurture further change talk
"It takes a lot of time to check everything before I can leave my apartment."	"You waste a lot of time. And you have more important priorities than checking."	"So, it's time-consuming and you sound frustrated with that. You might not like having to spend your time that way."
I don't sleep well, and I'm often tired at work the next day. It makes it hard to focus on what needs to get done."	"I can see how that would really be a problem. And if this doesn't get resolved, it could affect other areas as well. Maybe it will even put your job at risk."	"So, you've noticed that your concentration is affected. And it sounds like that might create some problems at work. Can you say more about that?"
"I want to be normal— not so crazy with anxiety all the time."	"So, that's really important. Change might be hard, but it's definitely worth it if you feel less abnormal."	"One thing that could be good about changing is that you might not feel so alone—maybe you'll feel a little less deviant, less ashamed."
"I get so anxious talking to people. So, I don't have a lot of friends."	"And you can't spend the rest of your life being alone. You have to get more comfortable with people."	"The anxiety makes it hard to make friends. And I'm guessing that sometimes that can be lonely."

about change that still feel foreign or threatening. This is especially true early on, when the change position is still fragile and the status quo position is still dominant. Again, in MI the arguments for change must come from the client, not the therapist. Alternatively, getting slightly underneath or behind initial change talk, and gently encouraging elaboration, feels safer to clients and is more productive in slowly and gently building elaboration of the merits of change.

Thus, while elaboration of change talk is an important goal in building the client's resolve to change, not all attempts to draw out, explore, or elaborate these arguments will be well received or effective in furthering that goal. It is important to stay connected with the underlying MI spirit, including reinforcing client authority, freedom from pressure to move toward change, creating an atmosphere of discovery and curiosity, and so on. Doing so is more likely to yield more gentle, less emphatic therapist reflections that stay closer to the client's experience and possible meaning.

ROLLING WITH RESISTANCE
WHEN ELABORATING CHANGE TALK

When clients more fully articulate desired directions (reasons to change) or limitations of existing ways of being (downsides of the status quo), they often "go back" or temporarily revisit the status quo position. This is a natural fluctuation in the process of exploring ambivalence. Just as clients find themselves articulating reasons to change—arguing or objecting to the status quo—when exploring resistance to change, they can also retreat to the status quo position when more fully articulating the reasons to change. That is, finding oneself saying aloud "This is really a problem," or "I'm really upset about the toll this is taking," or "This is not what I want for my life" internally encourages one to commit to the position. It exerts internal pressure to act or be in accordance with the stated view/position. That is, in the process of elaborating the change position, clients are repeatedly making arguments *to themselves* for change, and consequently they experience mounting or increasing pressure to change. While increasing such internal advocacy and momentum for change in the client is the goal in MI, given the potential of this process to retreat to the status quo position, it is important to be prepared to roll with resistance in this process.

The process of resolving ambivalence, and elaborating reasons for change, is typically far from a linear one (i.e., one often examines reasons to change and then reasons to not change). Consequently, the therapist takes opportunities to elaborate emergent change talk and evokes such contemplation of the change position while continually listening for and being prepared to roll with resistance upon the reemergence of the status quo position. That is, just as a therapist should not persist in examining the benefits of staying the same if the client is articulating significant change talk, the therapist should also not insist on elaborating change talk in the face of significant resistance to change.

Take opportunities to elaborate change talk while continually being prepared to roll with resistance.

Moving between these two positions (often quickly) characterizes therapeutic work at this stage. Thus, rolling with resistance is an important skill in helping the client continue to envision and elaborate the change position. For example, in the process of elaborating the change position, a client with PTSD might say, "I really want to be more happy. I'm so tired of living in this constant state of being on guard about being attacked again. And I know it's possible. (*pause*) But it's just so hard. It's so automatic to get sucked back into being afraid." Sometimes quickly rolling with such resistance (e.g., validating that "it is hard to change—you're absolutely right!") or reinforcing autonomy ("Sounds like there might be some good reasons to change, but only you can know whether it's worth the effort") or double-sided reflection ("There are some good arguments for changing, but it sure isn't easy") can resolve the concern and effectively move the client back to elaborating the change position (see Chapter 12 for a more detailed discussion of rolling with resistance). If resistance to change persists, the therapist can continue to roll with this resistance until change talk reemerges.

FURTHER WAYS TO ELABORATE CHANGE TALK

Sometimes more structured activities or exercises can also be useful in helping clients envision the arguments favoring change and immerse themselves more fully in considering the change position. Below, I present two such optional exercises that can supplement the skills already discussed for evoking and elaborating change talk. These include writing letters envisioning the future under conditions of change and no change and the use of a role play to help clients inhabit, articulate, and respond from the change position. However, these exercises are typically useful only when the client has begun to articulate significant change talk and the therapist is seeking to consolidate this. In the absence of significant levels of change talk, the exercises can risk engendering resistance. Note that these exercises are entirely optional, and a therapist can effectively work on fully elaborating change talk without them. And, consistent with MI spirit, these exercises should always be suggested as possibilities that clients are totally free to either accept or decline, whichever they prefer.

Letters Envisioning the Future

In a variant on the task of looking forward, clients can be invited to consider writing two letters to themselves as a possible between-sessions task: envisioning the future with and without their anxiety/depression (i.e., under conditions of change and no change). These can serve as evocative tools to further develop client exploration and elaboration of, respectively, the downsides to the status quo and the benefits to change. Once the client has begun to articulate and elaborate change talk, the exercise is especially useful in immersing the client in the contemplation of change, typically eliciting a large amount of change talk.

Specifically, the client is invited to consider writing two letters, addressed to him- or herself and dated 1 year from today (or whatever reference point in the future would be "be a time for reflection on your life"). In the first letter, the client writes about what life would be like if he or she made a 180-degree turn and decided to change. For the purpose of this exercise, the client can ignore the how-to's for now and just imagine that he or she has been very successful in making the change, and it worked out very well. The client is to reflect back on the year and describe in detail what is different and how he or she feels about these changes (e.g., "Do people treat you differently?," "Do you treat yourself differently?," "Do you have opportunities you didn't have before?," "Do you do things you didn't do before?," "Are there changes in the way you are with others?," "How are others reacting to the change, and how are their lives different because you have changed?"). The client can also be encouraged to describe in detail how he or she *feels* about each of those changes. If the changes are important, the therapist describes how and why they are significant.

In the second letter, the client writes about how life would be 1 year from now (or whatever reference point has been selected) if nothing changed and imagining the worst possible outcome of that. In other words, "If life a year from now were exactly the same as now, what would that look like exactly? How would that feel? How do you feel as you reflect back on another year with the anxiety and mood troubles? What else has changed or gotten worse? How do you feel about yourself, others, your future, and the like)? What kinds of things are you missing out on, and how important is that to you—and how do you feel about that?"

If the client decides to complete the letters, he or she may read them aloud in the session, if they prefer, or simply comment in session on their discoveries and the impact of the exercise. This material could then again be processed with a view to elaborating the important perceived consequences under conditions of, first, change and then no change.

Consider the following session excerpt of MI with a married woman with agoraphobia and panic disorder who completed this task:

CLIENT: I guess maybe it's been in the back of my mind, but I tried not to think about it. It really came to light when I started to write those letters we talked about last week—you know, if I remained anxious and then if I didn't remain anxious. I only projected 2 years from now . . . but I hope that within 2 years I'm going to be able to at least do a little bit of traveling. But when I was writing that letter and what my life might be like if I remained anxious, I thought, "You know, I wonder what this might be like for Mike [her husband]." (*Starts crying . . . long pause.*) I think as much as you love a person, you can only take so much. And I think that someday, maybe, he's going to sort of get tired of waiting around for me to say "Hey, maybe I can go somewhere today." (*tearful*) And I know if I said that to him he would be upset and say that's not true. But I'm sure that if I . . . if my anxiety stays the way it is at times, he's going to be going places by himself (*long pause*), and I don't really think that's how he pictured his life.

THERAPIST: Whether or not it means him actually leaving you, you really could see him being very hurt by not getting to do things with you. He's been pretty patient, pretty understanding so far, but your worry is that if this were to continue, this could really hurt him. (*pause*) And I can see that that's really important to you.

CLIENT: Yes! Having a good healthy marriage (*tearful*) . . . Mike's feelings . . . his happiness . . . mean a lot to me.

Role Play

Another optional exercise to immerse the client in more fully elaborating the change position is the use of a role play. Again, this is entirely optional and not necessary to accomplishing the goal of strengthening and elaborating change talk, but the exercise may be useful to some. As with any MI intervention or suggestion, sensitivity to client engagement and resistance is critical.

Here, the therapist can play the role of articulating the arguments for the status quo position that the client has discovered and/or the common objections that arise (or might arise) when the client considers taking steps to change (e.g., "I don't know that thinking more positively makes sense. What if something happens—and, trust me, it has—and then you're unprepared," or "You know, it may be better to not risk attracting the attention of others. It's so hard to deal with criticism. It's bound to end badly and might not be worth the risk"). The client's task is to respond to these by counterarguing (to defeat the therapist; e.g., "Well, my experience has been that anticipating the worst hasn't helped me to better deal with the bad stuff that happens. I just get anxious anyway," or "It's not for certain that it will end badly. And it fits better with what I really want to be like—more open").

If the client struggles a bit, the therapist can coach the client through this process by validating the difficulty of the task and encouraging the client to just brainstorm possible responses. Alternatively, the therapist can temporarily switch roles to illustrate the client's task. It is also useful to start with relatively easier or less persuasive arguments for the status quo, versus beginning with arguments that are likely to feel more powerful and persuasive to the client (leading him or her to shut down). You might even ask the client before the task about "What could I say that would really be hard to argue against?" After the exercise, you could debrief the client by asking him or her what the experience was like, what stood out in the exercise, which arguments were especially hard to counter, what statements resonated the most in the responses he or she made, and so on. This can further illuminate important arguments for change that resonate with the client and illuminate arguments that still have the power to get in the way of change (that could then be explored more fully by using the skills on navigating resistance to change that were presented in Chapter 6).

SUMMARY

It is important for the therapist to develop a sensitivity to recognizing or hearing "change talk" (arguments in favor of change and against the status quo) since such talk indicates that the client has shifted to or is currently occupying the change position. Accordingly, when this occurs, the therapist uses a combination of questions and reflections (sensitively delivered to not be beyond the client's experience and meaning) that prompt and invite him or her to further elaborate this position. Regardless of whether such arguments in favor of change spontaneously emerge or are evoked by the therapist, it is important to gently help the client work toward strengthening the change position, which initially is often quite fragile. In doing so, it is also important to be prepared to hear, integrate, work with, and roll with the status quo position (which often objects to such serious contemplation of change). Helping the client get in touch with and more fully elaborate his or her inherent and most authentic values is a key ally for the client in the process of envisioning change and resisting the powerful forces of the status quo. In the next chapter, systematically developing value–behavior discrepancies that help the client further increase his or her resolve for change is discussed.

8

⁂

Developing Discrepancy

Once you have helped the client achieve a fuller understanding of the forces for and against change and a greater awareness of authentically valued life directions, opportunities arise to systematically further the development of discrepancy between these positions. Systematically identifying discrepancies between what the client intrinsically desires and values, on the one hand (what gives, or would give, his or her life meaning), and current behavior that is inhibiting or inconsistent with those directions, on the other, helps to build the client's resolve to change. Developing such discrepancies is one of the core principles of MI.

Some of this important work on developing discrepancy occurs through identifying incentives for change that are meaningful and emotional and that impinge on important client values (discussed in the preceding chapter). Therapists can also further extend such work by both evoking and actively identifying and reflecting value–behavior discrepancies to bring these to the client's attention. The therapist working within the MI spirit does so in order to invite and enable clients to wrestle with and resolve such discrepancies. In this chapter, after briefly discussing the importance of value–behavior discrepancies, I describe and illustrate various ways of systematically developing such discrepancies in the service of building client resolve for change.

WHY VALUE–BEHAVIOR DISCREPANCIES
ARE IMPORTANT

We know from research in social psychology that heightening awareness of our values promotes value-consistent behavior (Festinger, 1957). That is, we strive for consistency between our behavior and our beliefs and values. Thus, there is a natural pull when dissonance between these arises and we are then motivated to seek resolution to such value–behavior discrepancies. The dissonance that arises upon realizing that one is not being consistent with one's values can be resolved by either reevaluating or reducing the significance of the value or producing behavior consistent with the value. Clients will often pull their behavior in line with their stated values, since it is typically much more difficult to devalue something of importance

It's harder to change values to line up with behavior than the reverse.

than it is to change one's behavior to be consistent with a cherished value. This process often requires patience (from both therapist and client) since it can be difficult and often jarring for clients to realize that they are not behaving consistently with their values and to ponder solutions for reconciling these discrepancies.

Systematically attending to and developing such inconsistencies for the client to consider heightens such dissonance and promotes efforts to attain greater consistency. Consider the example in the preceding chapter of the young mother with depression who realized that her depression was hurting her children. Having identified a critically important value and a meaningful life direction for the client (being a good mother), the therapist sought to increase awareness of the pain and costs of the depression in light of those values and the obstacles the depression presented to the client in achieving her goals. In some sense, then, realizing and experiencing the toll the depression took on her parenting created a "problem" for her in that it represented a discrepancy from important values that in turn pulled for resolution.

Thus, the therapist strives to help clients bring their values into the foreground by using reflective listening to highlight discrepancies between these and the anxious/depressed position. For example:

- "It's important to you to live your own life; yet, you keep trying to please others."
- "Worrying about staying healthy seems to be making you sick."
- "You value being a skilled professional, but your anxiety prevents you from consulting with colleagues and attending continuing education events."
- "Worrying is a way of getting control; yet, I also hear it makes you feel out of control."

Inviting clients to consider and reflect on these discrepancies facilitates intrinsic motivation and can create significant momentum for change.

EVOKING DISCREPANCY

One relatively straightforward way of developing discrepancy is to have the client assess the degree to which existing beliefs and behaviors are effective in achieving what he or she inherently desires and values. For example: "You mentioned needing to feel closer to others; to what degree is the anxiety helping with that important goal?," or "One of the things that has emerged for you is a sense of wanting to enjoy life more and have more peace of mind. To what degree is the worry/checking/planning/perfectionism helping you with that?," or "Preparing a lot—like going over your notes many times and doing copious amounts of reading—is intended to help you be a better teacher. What grade would you give those things in accomplishing that?"

You could also use rating scales to help with this exploration, for example, "Rate how effective X (the existing way of being) is on a scale of 1, not at all effective, to 10, extremely effective." Then you can also explore the client's ratings to further develop change talk, for example, "It's helping at a 5 out of 10. Why a 5 and not a 10? Tell me about the part of you that doubts that it's entirely effective." Thus, the therapist can have the client generate discrepancies by asking about or evoking them.

The Spirit behind Developing Discrepancy

Importantly, developing value–behavior discrepancies is done in the spirit of preserving client autonomy and not in a spirit of "confronting" the client, correcting him or her, or insisting on change, since these latter responses stem from a therapist-as-expert attitude. That is, the MI therapist's interest in evoking such discrepancies, for example, is not to "prove" to the client something that the therapist already knows to be true (i.e., that these existing ways of being don't work). Rather, the MI therapist works to systematically increase awareness of value–behavior discrepancies so that the client can reflect on and wrestle with these for him- or herself, free from pressure to make conclusions favoring change. It is up to the client to resolve such discrepancies, with the therapist's role involving evoking and noticing them, bringing them to the client's attention (in a nonjudgmental manner), and supporting the client in his or her efforts to resolve these and envision alternative means of living consistently with one's values (if the client decides that the behavior needs to change).

To illustrate, if the client responds to the therapist's attempt to evoke discrepancy by concluding that the anxiety is relatively ineffective in

> *Developing discrepancies is done in the spirit of preserving client autonomy, not to confront the client.*

achieving desired goals, the MI therapist's response does not reflect an attitude of "I told you so" or "I knew it, and now you see it too." Rather, the therapist's role is to note whether the client responds with further change talk (in which case this is reflected and further elaborated) or resistance to change (in which case the therapist rolls with resistance until change talk reemerges).

Below I demonstrate MI-inconsistent and MI-consistent responses when the therapist seeks to evoke discrepancy.

THERAPIST: And how effective would you say that getting reassurance is in helping you with this important goal of feeling more relaxed—being less anxious about your health?

CLIENT: At the time, I do feel better when I go to the doctor and he reassures me that he can't find anything wrong. But it doesn't last very long.

THERAPIST: [MI inconsistent response] That's right. You see, the anxiety promises that you will feel less anxious if you seek reassurance, but what we know is that it actually makes you more anxious rather than less.

THERAPIST: [MI consistent response] I see. So, even though it seems to help, it doesn't last. And how important is that limitation of reassurance to you?

or

THERAPIST: [MI consistent response] So, based on your experience, getting reassurance may not work in the long run. And this may or may not be of interest to you, but that also fits with what we know about reassurance—that it can actually keep the anxiety going in the long run.

NOTICING AND REFLECTING DISCREPANCIES

In addition to evoking discrepancies, the therapist can play an active role in both being alert for and noticing such discrepancies of existing ways of being with core values and bringing them to the client's attention for further consideration. Such opportunities can often arise in the context of helping the client to more fully elaborate his or her values. Consider the following two examples of the therapist identifying value–behavior discrepancies in this context and bringing these to the client's attention.

This first example is in the context of working with a young man with social anxiety.

THERAPIST: What would you like to be like in social situations?

CLIENT: I really admire people who can just be themselves—like, be relaxed in conversations . . . be spontaneous . . . just speak about what's on their minds . . . whatever that might be. I don't do that. I stick to safe stuff like my accomplishments . . . what I do.

THERAPIST: Yeah. So, that's the kind of person you would like to be . . . in the moment . . . just saying whatever is there right now without thinking about where it's going or that it has to go somewhere.

CLIENT: Right. Like just being true to whatever I'm thinking and speaking from that.

THERAPIST: So, you value being authentic, yet you find yourself being dishonest. Rather than putting yourself out there and being real, the anxiety has you put on this pretense . . . this kind of mask . . . based on what it thinks other people want to see.

CLIENT: (pause) I have a knot in my stomach right now with what you just said.

THERAPIST: Say more.

CLIENT: I'm being fake. I'm not being authentic.

THERAPIST: And that hurts you.

CLIENT: Very much. (pause) Like another thing I really take pride in is being a model or mentor for others . . . an example that they can follow. Like, with my students I get such joy out of seeing them flourish and learn. I'm just myself when I teach, you know . . . relaxed.

THERAPIST: And you'd really like to be more like that. And I'm guessing that one of things you don't want to teach your students is how to pretend with others . . . how to hide . . . how to pull off this pretense.

CLIENT: Absolutely not.

THERAPIST: That's important. (pause) It seems that you might be modeling the opposite of what you really believe when you do that. Things like "What others think is more important than what you think". . . . "You should always try to please people and get them to like you."

CLIENT: I don't agree with that at all. That's no way to live.

THERAPIST: So, you're not living as long as this pretense is in place. You're safe in a way . . . You're protected . . . but you're not who you need and want to be.

CLIENT: (*pause*) Oh, man, I'm going to work on that one.

This next illustration involves a young woman with a highly deferential interpersonal style who was recounting an incident in which her mother was quite neglectful of her needs. In particular, her mother invited the family of her brother's new fiancé to dinner on her birthday. This left the client feeling angry and hurt and perpetuated a chronic feeling of being invisible, unrecognized, and dismissed by others. An opportunity to develop discrepancy arose later when she was exploring her values in relationships.

THERAPIST: It sounds like you are a very caring person. Someone who really values being there for others.

CLIENT: Right. I think that's just the right thing to do in relationships. I think it's important to do things for others, to be there for others, to try to understand them.

THERAPIST: So, this fits with your values in relationships. It's important to be there for others—it makes for meaningful connections with others, for good relationships.

CLIENT: Right. Like, when you try to understand someone—are there for them—they'll be there for you when you need that.

THERAPIST: I see. A kind of reciprocity. In other words, you can't expect someone to be there for you if you aren't there for them.

CLIENT: Exactly.

THERAPIST: That makes sense. At the same time, I hear that it doesn't always work out that way with your mom. You value working hard to be there for her so that she'll be there for you. But instead she lets you down when you need her.

CLIENT: (*long pause*) To be honest. It doesn't work out that way in a lot of my relationships.

THERAPIST: Yikes. So, all the effort you're expending to please other people in order to have good relationships may not be paying off so well. You might need to consider a different way of operating or investing your energy. Is that right?

As these examples illustrate, realization of failure to live consistently with one's values is uncomfortable and painful. Such discrepancies, when noticed and brought to the client's attention, pull for resolution in order to reestablish consistency between what one genuinely needs and wants, and behavior to meet those important needs (needs of which the client may have previously been only dimly aware). And striving to actualize one's values can serve as a catalyst for behavior change.

> *Realization of failure to live up to one's values is uncomfortable—and pulls for resolution.*

Often, upon the contemplation of such discrepancies, clients begin to more actively consider and prepare for change. For example, consider the following response upon realizing an important discrepancy in a client with agoraphobia.

THERAPIST: When we think about those advantages—so many of those things that you do are coming from this sense of caring for people. On the one hand, a lot of this stuff—staying at home, avoiding—is to care. But now there's also this feeling that that caring could end up hurting a lot of people—caring in that way. That you are going about trying to do something very good—to not have people hurt, to not lose people—and yet out of all that is this potential to hurt other people, and yourself. What do you make of that?

CLIENT: I guess I'm going about it all the wrong way—showing people how I care about them (*pause*). And that I need to take some risks—as scary as it might be.

Living consistently with one's values is also very challenging, since it often means going against others' expectations or familiar, habitual ways of being that often underlie and perpetuate anxiety and depression. Thus, in the context of MI spirit, therapists can help support clients in working through the challenges of envisioning what living a value-consistent life would look like and in dealing with the difficulties that will arise when taking steps to do so. These challenges are nicely articulated by a client who was chronically perfectionist and highly achievement-oriented.

CLIENT: I see now that there is a part of me that knows what I want and what I should do. And when I hear that and follow that, I feel better. But it's hard to hear that.

THERAPIST: To really allow yourself to be yourself. Absolutely. What's hard about it?

CLIENT: It goes against everything I've ever done and believed. Like, my whole life I have been driven by the mentality of "set goals, take steps, plan your future so that you can achieve." And now I see that that was never really what I pictured for myself. It doesn't make me feel good. (*pause*) I'm almost embarrassed to say this, but what I really want is to be a good wife and mother.

THERAPIST: To invest yourself in something that really matters to you.

CLIENT: Yeah. I feel like that is what I am here for. That is what I most want to do. Like, I really value my marriage and even being a good doggie mom. I really care for others well. And I think I could be a great nurse and a great mom too.

THERAPIST: And when you say that, you seem to feel good. It feels right. But it sure is hard to admit that, because then you might have to start "walking the talk."

CLIENT: Yes. Like, when I listen to myself, that is what I want. But I wish I were different too and I wanted different things. Like, it's not okay in our society to say "I want to be a mom."

THERAPIST: So, part of the conflict is that you see where you need to go, but if you go there, others might not approve, you might not fit in.

CLIENT: Exactly. Like, ever since I was a little girl, my mom wanted me to be a lawyer. And I would say to my grandmother, "I think I want to be a nurse." And I never really felt that I had the option, because I was the one everyone was counting on to succeed—to really make it.

THERAPIST: You had to meet their expectations. You couldn't disappoint them. You had to be what they needed you to be instead of what you wanted to be. And if you don't do that anymore, maybe they won't respect you, maybe they won't care for you anymore. Is that right?

WHEN NOT CHANGING
IS CONSISTENT WITH ONE'S VALUES

As we have seen, the status quo position is often inconsistent with authentically valued life directions and client values, and it thwarts the pursuit of these. But in other ways the status quo position can also be consistent with the client's core values. Accordingly, clients can fear that changing means losing important aspects of themselves or critical aspects of identity that the status quo helped actualize. That is, they can feel that, if they give up existing ways of being, they will also be giving up important means of expressing core values such as being caring, responsible, reliable, loving, and the like. At these times, clients can need help to envision alternative means of expressing these values and living consistently with them, free of the problem behavior.

For example, consider the following illustration of work with a woman suffering with depression who was beginning to realize that she desired more happiness in her life and this was an important goal for her. Yet, she also valued being helpful and available to others, being someone they could count on. Being reliable and helpful was a major way that she got esteem from her family in the past, and this played a significant role in her lifelong pattern of serving others and deferring to their needs.

CLIENT: I'm almost afraid to be happy.

THERAPIST: Say more. What's scary about it?

CLIENT: Well, because there are others who aren't happy. It's selfish to focus on your own happiness when others are suffering.

THERAPIST: You would feel guilty if you looked after myself.

CLIENT: Yes! I always feel like my job is to look after everyone else—be the surrogate mother.

THERAPIST: So, you can't just give yourself permission to be happy, because then you would be giving up something else that's important—helping others. I don't know if this fits for you at all, but in a way you are saying "If I'm happy, I can't be helpful."

CLIENT: Yeah. (pause) But that's not really true, is it—or at least it doesn't have to be.

THERAPIST: Just because you're happy, it doesn't mean that you stop caring. Is that what you mean?

CLIENT: Yeah, and maybe I can be even more effective in helping others if I'm happier.

THERAPIST: So, if I'm hearing you right, "helping others" sounds like it's important to you and you don't want to do anything to jeopardize that. But now you're thinking that "maybe I don't have to stay miserable to do that. In fact, maybe I can care for others better if I'm happier. Be more available to them." How does that sound to you? Do you believe that?

CLIENT: Yes, because since I've been depressed I find I'm just not available to others anymore, I don't want to be around anyone. And then I feel guilty about that!

THERAPIST: Wow! So, maybe looking after yourself, in a way, is the best thing you can do for others.

CLIENT: And for myself—because I really want to be happy.

THERAPIST: So, you've denied yourself happiness but you really think that it's something that you want and need now, and something that could also fit with your need to care for others.

DEVELOPING DISCREPANCY BY BRINGING THE TWO SIDES OF AMBIVALENCE TOGETHER

Another useful way to develop discrepancy is to simply bring together, or help the client simultaneously consider, his or her reasons for the status quo and the reasons for change. That is, after you have helped the client develop an understanding of both sides of the dilemma surrounding change, it can be useful to systematically bring these together. This may or may not involve client values, but nonetheless the activity invites clients to wrestle with the discrepancies and contradictions in these competing agendas. For example, if a pro (advantage) to staying the same was "It's easier" and cons included evidence of how anxiety creates problems for the person, the therapist might pull these together and ask for clarification. For example, "I'm wondering if you can help me sort something out. On the one hand, I hear you saying that staying the same is easier—less hassle. Yet, at the same time, it seems to make a lot of things harder because it's distracting and you can't concentrate. How do those fit together? I'm confused about whether it's really easier or not." Or "Avoiding allows you to not have to be anxious, and that sounds really useful. Somehow, though, you are still experiencing anxiety all the time. How does that fit together?"

> *Setting forth both sides of the client's ambivalence invites him or her to wrestle with the contradictions between them.*

Or "When you isolate yourself, you feel better, but I'm also hearing that it makes you feel worse. What's your sense of that?"

An alternative and more extended and systematic way of bringing both sides of the ambivalence together is to personify the two sides of the ambivalence and work toward establishing a dialogue between them. In this way, the client can develop a new perspective on change that is informed by both incentives for change rooted in client values (change position) and an understanding of the needs, beliefs, and fears being expressed by the part of the self that resists change (the status quo position).

In their book on ambivalence in psychotherapy, Engle and Arkowitz (2006) nicely illustrate the use of a two-chair approach developed and adapted from Gestalt therapy by Leslie Greenberg (2002) as a method for working through and resolving ambivalence about change. In this approach, the therapist helps the client personify and then speak from each position in order to facilitate understanding and experiential awareness of each perspective. Important discrepancies between current ways of being, on the one hand, and client values and needs, on the other, can become heightened in this approach.

Consider the use of a version of this approach to resolve ambivalence about change in work with a client who experienced debilitating performance anxiety and perfectionism. The client noted intense and chronic urges toward being extremely driven and in fact described herself as a "Class A workaholic." She felt incapable of any kind of self-care, downtime, or of saying "No" to colleagues' requests. She experienced strong feelings of guilt and internal pressure to continually improve her knowledge base in order to prove her worth and stave off pervasive feelings of inadequacy. She recognized the futility of these efforts in alleviating her anxiety, and in fact she was very frustrated with herself since she was well aware that she increasingly valued being able to relax and strongly desired more serenity and happiness in her life. Yet, she reported an extremely strong urge to persist with her "old" behaviors and demonstrated intense fear of relinquishing them.

Although I did not have the client alternate between sitting in two different chairs, I helped her conceptualize and inhabit these two positions separately by suggesting that we specify different names for these competing perspectives on change. She chose to name the fearful aspect of herself "Workaholic Jane" (the status quo position), and the competing aspect of herself "Desired Jane" (the change position). Given that the status quo position was clearly stronger and dominating her behavior choices (i.e., was "more alive"), I asked the client to speak first from the perspective of Workaholic Jane. The dialogue proceeded as follows:

CLIENT: [speaking as Workaholic Jane] You're a fraud, and everyone will find out if you don't work extra hard to make sure they don't.

THERAPIST: You're scared that if you're not on the job you'll be humiliated, and that's extremely painful. Is that right? [empathic reflection inviting further elaboration]

CLIENT: Yes. I just want to crawl into the floor every time I screw up.

THERAPIST: It's *horribly* painful—devastating. And you fear that you can't afford to screw up. There's a lot on the line. [empathic reflection inviting further elaboration]

CLIENT: I'll be nothing—good for nothing. If I can't do this job—I have nothing. Everything I've worked so hard for all these years . . . *(tearful)*

THERAPIST: And you're also thinking, "what will everyone else think of me if I can't do this job?" [empathic reflection inviting further elaboration]

CLIENT: I can't even think about that.

THERAPIST: (*pause*) So, in a way, Workaholic Jane is trying to prevent disaster here. She may be tough at times and kind of critical and harsh, but she seems to have a good heart. She wants to spare you from this kind of suffering. Would that be right? [reframing resistance to change; highlighting the positive intentions behind the chronic workaholic pattern]

CLIENT: That's true. (*long pause*) She is kind of caring.

THERAPIST: What do you mean? Say more. [encouraging further elaboration of the positive reframing of the "problem"]

CLIENT: She's very passionate. She cares deeply about what happens to me.

THERAPIST: She looks out for you, in a way. She's very concerned. Fiercely protective, too, it sounds like. [empathic reflection encouraging further elaboration]

CLIENT: You know, as we're talking what's coming up is being bullied in college. I just remember that people always thought that, as a foreign student, I couldn't make it. I wasn't as good as them.

THERAPIST: And Workaholic Jane helped you with that—helped you prove that you could do it. In fact, she was a terrific ally in that fight. Sounds like someone you would definitely want in your corner. [continuing to identify the good things about the chronic workaholic pattern]

CLIENT: Yes. She pushed me to succeed—to always do better—be better.

THERAPIST: Sounds like she was a life saver at a critical time. She helped you to feel strong. And naturally she's terribly afraid that if you let go of that drive, if you let up, you'll be unprotected—you'll fall prey to the bullies that are out there waiting to pounce. [encouraging further understanding of the problem, more compassionate understanding of the behavior]

CLIENT: Yes. I'm terrified that, if I give in and let myself relax, I won't be successful in this job and lose everything I've worked for . . . my whole reputation.

THERAPIST: And I bet Workaholic Jane really resents Desired Jane. (*sarcastically*) Oh, yeah, "Just chill. Relax." Are you insane—there's a battle going on out there! If you let down your guard, you'll be crushed. [continuing empathic reflection, reframing]

CLIENT: That's exactly how it feels. (*pause*) But I know that's not true. [Change talk emerges.]

THERAPIST: You have a sense that it might be safe to let up a bit. That sounds like Desired Jane talking. Is that right?

CLIENT: Yes.

THERAPIST: What makes you suspect that it might be okay to let up a bit? [encouraging client to speak from the change, or Desired Jane, position]

CLIENT: [speaking as Desired Jane] I know that I'm actually more productive, not less, when I relax. And I really want to be happier. I'm just so miserable all the time. And, with all this anxiety, I just can't concentrate—can't focus. That's not helping me. It's hurting me. [More change talk emerges.]

THERAPIST: So, Workaholic Jane is well intentioned, but she tends to go overboard sometimes. And, if I'm hearing you right, she may not be right in how she sees the world. I don't know, I could be wrong about this, but it sounds a little bit like the rules have changed and no one told Workaholic Jane. [summary of the ambivalence, ending with what is most alive—change talk; also seeking to deepen this position by suggesting a possible alternative view that challenges the value of the status quo position]

CLIENT: (*silent but looking intently at the therapist*)

THERAPIST: In Workaholic Jane's world, everyone is a critic. Her students are out to get her. Her colleagues are out to get her. But I also hear the other part of you, Desired Jane, who seems to feel that that may not be the case, at least not all the time. That not everyone is a critic and if that's true, maybe you can relax a bit, be yourself more, and stop proving yourself all the time. Is that right?

CLIENT: (*smiling*) You know, I really am starting to suspect that other people are not out to get me. I really like some of my colleagues, and they're quite supportive. And I know in my heart that most students really enjoy my classes. They get a lot out of them. [further elaboration of the change position]

THERAPIST: And enjoy you as a teacher. You have a lot to offer. And I can totally see how that would be the case. Personally, from what you have told me and what I know of you, I have no doubt that the smart money is on you being a terrific teacher. If you were to speak from the perspective of Desired Jane, what would she tell Workaholic Jane? How would she help her relax? [affirmation; encouraging further elaboration of the change position and bringing the two sides together]

CLIENT: [speaking as Desired Jane] Thanks for keeping me on my toes. But I've got this. I'm good.

THERAPIST: You're saying, "You can trust me. Things won't fall apart." And what about what Desired Jane really values. Is there something that motivates her, other than fear? How does she get going in the morning?

CLIENT: You know, when I do it because I love it, I feel so much more motivated.

Notice how this way of working builds on the skills we have already discussed—namely, empathic reflection, understanding and reframing resistance to change (positive motivations underlying the status quo positions), encouraging compassionate understanding and acceptance of action tendencies and beliefs that frustrate the person (Chapter 6), as well as noticing emergent change talk and seeking to elaborate it (Chapter 7). Working in this way can further exploration and resolution of ambivalence by rendering discrepancies between the competing agendas (sides of the ambivalence) more salient. It also encourages interaction between the two sides and facilitates the development of a more harmonious, rather than antagonistic, way of relating. Finally, this approach can help the person begin to develop skills in responding to the status quo position based on his or her authentic values and desires (the change position).

Notice that in example above I also contributed a suggestion and offered a piece of advice ("What about thinking about it this way . . . ") that occurred to me in the context of this interaction. Bringing in suggestions that occur to you from this external frame of reference ("Try this," "What about this?") can be extremely useful if they are offered in the MI spirit of preserving client choice and autonomy. How to bring in your suggestions and expertise while preserving the MI spirit is the focus of the next chapter.

SUMMARY

Explicitly developing discrepancy between the client's authentic and inherently valued directions and incentives/arguments for change (the change position), on the one hand, and incentives/arguments supporting existing ways of being (the status quo position) can be very valuable in furthering client change talk and resolve to change. Such discrepancies often arouse discomfort, which therefore naturally helps promote resolution to establish consistency between one's beliefs and behavior. That is, it is important to us to behave consistently with what we intrinsically value. Becoming more aware of these values (which are often obscured in the face of unrelenting anxiety) naturally renders discrepancies with existing beliefs and behavior more salient and creates opportunities to further develop value–behavior discrepancies. The therapist can either seek to identify, be alert for, and reflect these or seek to evoke such discrepancies. In either case, the therapist working with MI aims to heighten the awareness of such discrepancies and encourage their resolution. As with all MI methods, inviting consideration of discrepancies of values with existing ways of being is done in the spirit of helping clients resolve these for themselves and supporting them in working through these often painful realizations.

PART IV

ભ

Extending Motivational Interviewing into the Action Phase

9
⌘

Evoking and Elaborating
Client Expertise

HOW MOTIVATIONAL INTERVIEWING
CAN INFORM ACTION-ORIENTED THERAPIES

When ambivalence is reduced or resolved, clients show signs of active preparation for and consideration of change. With increased resolve and motivation, clients often also spontaneously begin to take steps toward change. At this stage, there is often a palpable shift in the client, with greater interest in specifically envisioning change and experimenting with ways to achieve these desired changes. Essentially, the focus shifts from *why* to change to *how* to change.

When lower resistance to change and increased interest in achieving change are present, the therapist needs to shift with the client and support him or her in the process of planning for, experimenting with, and supporting the efforts to change. That is, the therapist needs to move from primarily or exclusively building resolve to change to supporting clients in envisioning and accomplishing specific steps to accomplish the changes they seek. Therapies that involve specific change strategies, methods, and techniques prove very useful to clients at this stage. And clients with higher levels of motivation or readiness for change welcome and engage quite readily with such approaches since they provide explicit guidance and direction for achieving relief from the noxious feelings associated with anxiety and depression, as well as structured assistance with the problems, issues, and ways of being that perpetuate them. That is, there is a synergy between clients who are ready for and wanting guidance on change and therapists who can bring to the fore their considerable expertise on specific methods to help them accomplish this. Clients with lower resistance and greater willingness to engage in treatment are likely to benefit the most from a wide variety of approaches that offer them a credible framework for changing and explicit guidance on how to do so.

Directive versus Supportive Methods of Facilitating Actions to Change

When clients show interest in acquiring and learning about specific ways of accomplishing change, therapists can naturally feel a need to shift to a more educational and directive approach. Underlying many action-oriented approaches is a particular set of assumptions, however. That is, clients are presumed to have particular deficits or dysfunctions. These deficits might include poor coping skills, maladaptive beliefs and cognitions, behavioral deficits such as withdrawal from pleasurable activities or avoidance of fear-provoking stimuli, or chronic maladaptive patterns of interaction or the like. The therapist then seeks to help the client identify and correct these deficits. Here, the therapist typically plays an active role in structuring, directing, providing information, and teaching clients healthier and more adaptive ways of being.

Accordingly, in many action-oriented approaches, the therapist is considered to have specific expertise that is offered to the client in the service of his or her recovery. And when adopted and implemented by the client, such experiences are considered central to advancing the client's recovery. Here, the therapist may be viewed (by him- or herself and the client) as having unique expertise that the client typically does not possess and that is currently unavailable to the client. From this perspective, the client's role is to integrate and implement this external expertise. While the importance of the relationship is clearly recognized in many action-oriented approaches, there is a strong emphasis on specific techniques (and therapist technical proficiency in administering these interventions) since they are considered to be the active ingredients of the approach, or mechanisms on which recovery is predicated.[1]

In contrast, as we have seen, the view of the therapy process underlying MI is quite different. In MI, the spirit or attitude underlying any therapist action is considered of paramount importance in influencing the effectiveness of any therapist offering, input, or intervention. And this spirit is considered more significant than particular techniques. This does not

---

[1] See Bohart and Tallman (1999) and Wampold (2001) for excellent and more detailed elaboration and evaluation of the assumptions underlying the medical and contextual models of conducting therapy.

mean that the techniques or specific therapist actions are unimportant or not needed in MI—quite the contrary. Rather, in MI there is an emphasis on "technique in context," that is, an awareness of and explicit attentiveness to the larger context in which therapist offerings are delivered and therapist actions take place. No technique or therapist action is devoid of context, and in MI key contextual parameters include client receptivity and engagement, the relationship between the client and the therapist, and the interpersonal or communicative significance of therapist actions (what they communicate about the therapist's view of the client and the process of change).

In MI there is an explicit emphasis on nurturing and cultivating a particular attitude or view of the client. While this underlying attitude or spirit was elaborated in Chapter 2, a central aspect of this view is the belief that clients have inherent expertise, not only to resolve ambivalence but also to initiate and accomplish change. That is, clients know more than they realize (or often give themselves credit for), and they can be relied upon, under the right conditions, to resolve the difficulties they are seeking relief from. Trusting this, the MI therapist is primarily concerned with creating a safe, collaborative space conducive to uncovering, discovering, calling forth, and helping clients realize and apply this inherent expertise. Thus, the therapist prioritizes client expertise (client-as-expert) over their own (therapist-as-expert).

Is there a role for this view in the action stage—when clients need to focus more on developing specific skills and action plans to accomplish change? I argue that the underlying spirit of MI (and the methods that flow from it) can be used as a foundational platform from which any specific change-oriented approach can be practiced. Integrating the foundational spirit and methods of MI has much to offer in terms of informing the *process* of therapy and facilitating sensitivity to the contextual influences (client receptivity, therapist attitude, etc.) inherent therein. Thus, infusing MI into the action stage of treatment is largely concerned with the context in which action is considered, conceptualized, planned, and implemented, and the promotion of sensitivity to these contextual factors.

Moreover, MI does not specify particular change strategies that should be used to achieve behavior change, but has much to say about the context in which such therapist inputs are offered. That is, integrating MI does not inform *what* techniques or methods of promoting change to use, but rather it can significantly inform *when* and *how* to support clients in selecting and implementing methods for achieving change. Here, therapists informed by MI can operate as guides or consultants to clients in developing, implementing, and processing their plans for change (Arkowitz & Burke, 2008; Rollnick, Miller, & Butler, 2008).

RECOGNIZING AND ELABORATING CLIENT EXPERTISE

Consistent with the view that clients possess inherent expertise with respect to problem resolution, the therapist infusing MI into treatment continuously searches for opportunities to evoke, build on, and work with this expertise. Doing so not only makes it more likely that the client will implement planned steps to change (since the actions to change were derived from them) but also represents important opportunities to build client self-efficacy and support previously unrecognized capabilities for self-determination. As noted by Rogers (1961): "It is the client who knows what hurts, what directions to go, what problems are crucial, what experiences have been deeply buried. It began to occur to me that unless I had a need to demonstrate my own cleverness and learning, I would do better to rely upon the client for the direction of movement in the process." This belief the therapist has in the client's inherent expertise—and the opportunity to search for this and explore and present these thoughts and ideas—helps clients realize that they can trust their own judgment and internal direction, that they do not need to defer to others' expertise but have inherent resources and wisdom they can draw on again and again, even after therapy has ended.

Therapists working with MI to help clients take action to change first evocatively seek to elicit client ideas and thoughts about how to proceed with taking action to change, prior to contributing their own. Clients can often be quick to defer to therapist expertise (perhaps consistent with previous experiences with other helpers that submission to the superior knowledge of the helper is expected, necessary, and desirable). And infusing MI into treatment means resisting this client deference in favor of preferentially eliciting and prioritizing client expertise. Failing to elicit client preferences, ideas, potential action steps and solutions, or quickly presenting the therapist's preferred approach, can send the message that therapist expertise is more important than client expertise and that the client should defer to this.

> *Presenting your preferred approach and neglecting the client's sends the message that your expertise is more important than the client's.*

This chapter considers opportunities for systematically eliciting client expertise in the context of helping clients with anxiety and related problems of depression take steps toward change. In particular, elaboration and illustration of this process in several common treatment situations is considered, including:

- Developing an action plan.
- Conceptualizing experiments with change.

- Processing efforts to change.
- Helping clients answer their own questions.

Of course, opportunities to elicit client expertise are not limited to these specific situations, and the therapist infusing MI into treatment seeks to systematically and preferentially elicit client expertise whenever possible. In this process, the therapist builds on and helps to develop client ideas but also contributes his or her own. Here, therapist suggestions and expertise are very important additions to the client's ideas and are offered to help shape and build on the client's existing ideas and preferences. The process is very much a collaborative effort, with each person contributing expertise on potential action steps and solutions. While eliciting client ideas and preferences is the primary focus of this chapter, the next chapter more fully elaborates effective ways of sharing your own valuable ideas and expertise in an MI-consistent manner.

Developing an Action Plan

In my experience, most clients with anxiety and depression are not typically lacking in knowledge of what to do to change. For example, when I ask clients with phobias what they would recommend to someone who has a phobia about dogs and wants to overcome it, the vast majority of clients recommend some form of graded exposure (e.g., "Get a puppy," "Be around a nice dog"). Similarly, clients with depression may be quite aware that oversleeping, overeating (or undereating), and withdrawal further negatively impact their mood. And clients are often painfully aware of what it is they "need to do" (e.g., be more assertive, not drink so much). It is rare for clients, in my experience, to have no ideas about what needs to change and how to go about accomplishing those changes.

Thus, most clients who have resolved to take action can often, when prompted, envision specific potentially useful steps for problem resolution. Thus, taking an approach that trusts, prizes, promotes, and relies heavily on client expertise about how to change essentially lets clients discover *for themselves* the value of solutions that most therapists are already familiar with. Moreover, this approach also has the advantage of considering solutions that the therapist had not considered. Over the years, one thing that has consistently impressed me is client creativity in developing plans and action steps to change. And often such solutions are far more creative than anything I could have come up with.

> *Clients who have resolved to take action often envision specific steps for problem resolution.*

In fact, if you ask clients how they might go about accomplishing change and they respond with "I don't know," this may be an indicator of lack of readiness to take such steps (i.e., "You are asking me to commit to something—taking action—for which I am not ready"). Alternatively, such a response may also be communicating important information about how clients view the process of therapy and your/their role, or how they view their role with others more generally (as one of submission and deference). That is, clients may tend to view the therapist/others as the expert and may discount their own expertise. In these cases, it can be worthwhile to provide information about the collaborative process of therapy and its reliance on clients' active involvement. For example:

"Unfortunately, I'm not that good where I can solve people's problems for them. I do have some expertise on what's worked with other people and what the research indicates and I'll certainly offer guidance and specific suggestions, exercises and ideas for you to consider as we work together. However, you are the best expert on yourself, and so we'll be drawing on your expertise a lot in this process and getting your feedback about how we're doing since only you know what makes the most sense or is the most helpful way of tackling this problem. That may be tough for you at times, I suspect, but treatment tends to work best, in my experience, if I try to help you figure out what *you* would like to do."

Evoking Action Steps

Table 9.1 contains a number of questions and prompts to evoke client ideas about possible steps to achieve change that can form the basis and/or the beginning of a change plan. Some of these have been drawn from Miller and Rollnick's (2002) suggestions for planning change and enhancing confidence. These have been supplemented with other possibilities for evocatively helping clients with anxiety and related problems envision steps to change.

Here, you are evoking the client's specific ideas about likely paths to the problem's resolution. Such an approach encourages clients to think about the steps they foresee to resolving the problem and demonstrates the therapist's interest in and respect for these ideas. The client's responses also provide important information about his or her beliefs about necessary treatment tasks and processes. The therapist can then use this to inform the treatment plan and tailor treatment to the client. Moreover, this process enables the therapist to elicit and build on the client's existing efforts since clients who have resolved to change often start taking steps to experiment with this. Both helpful/successful and unhelpful/unsuccess-

TABLE 9.1. Prompts for Eliciting Possible Action Steps

- "If you could picture a time in the future when this problem will be solved, what would have happened to bring that about?"
- "You like the idea of changing X . . . or being more Y. Where would be a good place to begin?"
- "If you and I were developing a plan for change for someone else who was exactly like you, what would you recommend?"
- "What steps have you already taken to change?"
- "When you have faced difficult changes in the past, what has helped? Is there anything from those experiences that might be relevant or potentially useful here?"
- "There may not be many, if any, but at times when you are less anxious, what are you doing or thinking that's different from the anxious times?" Or "When you are less depressed, what's different? How are you acting or thinking differently at those times?"
- "What makes the problem worse—and therefore, what might make it better?"
- "If you were to speak from that part of you that knows what you really want your life to be like, what would that person recommend as possibly helpful steps to get there?"

Use of scaling/rulers

> THERAPIST: Where would you say you are right now on this problem on a scale of 1 to 10, with 1 being "at my worst point" and 10 being "where I would ideally like to be"?
>
> CLIENT: Three.
>
> THERAPIST: How did you get from 1 to 3? [eliciting current action that has been helpful]

and

> THERAPIST: How might you go from a 3 to a 5? [eliciting possible future actions] or, If you pictured yourself at a 5 in the future, how would you have gotten there?

ful efforts are potentially informative in this regard. And mining these instances for information on precisely what was helpful, how the client did it, and how he or she managed to overcome the obstacles inherent in making change can be a useful springboard to enhancing client confidence in making change.

Consistent with MI spirit, freeing the client from pressure to automatically adopt the ideas (simply because he or she has articulated them) is important in facilitating the client's creative brainstorming about options. For example, a therapist can ask a client to envision, *hypothetically*, what steps one would take to resolve a specific problem the client has identified. For example, if the client has identified insomnia as a problem he or she would like to address, the therapist could ask, "What about us putting our heads together to generate ideas about how one might go about reducing insomnia—free from any pressure to act on these ideas. That is, you don't have to run out and implement any of these suggestions. Let's first get your thoughts and make a list of possibilities. We can examine them later to see whether any of them makes sense or would be worth trying. For now, let's just see what we come up with. How does that sound?" Such an approach is more commonly used in facilitating problem solving, since the pressure to take action can inhibit creativity. This way of working is also quite consistent with the noncoercive spirit of MI and can reduce evoking the resistance to change (obstacles, reasons to not take the step) that can often emerge when clients begin to more specifically envision how to change.

The therapist also plays an important role in supplementing the client's ideas. Again, any therapist contributions are offered in a spirit of supporting client autonomy, for example, "In addition, I also had some thoughts about things you might consider adding if they make sense to you. You know yourself best, so you are in the best position to determine the timing of these or whether they would be worth trying. Would you like to hear these?" Whether autonomy is explicitly preserved like this or only implicitly communicated by the therapist, the client is regarded as the ultimate arbiter on decisions about the methods, timing, and preferred actions toward change, with the therapist operating as a consultant to the client's change plans. In short, the therapist's ideas about specific exercises or action steps are very useful; it's a matter of timing and presenting them in an atmosphere that is free from coercion and pressure to change or to adopt the therapist's suggestions (see Chapter 10 for further elaboration on MI-informed ways of sharing and integrating therapist expertise).

Nurturing Change Talk

Once clients begin this process of specifically envisioning how to change, therapists assist them in further elaborating their ideas, evaluating the pros and cons of the options, and guiding them to develop specific experiments to test their ideas. The MI skills discussed previously in elaborating and nurturing change talk (see Chapter 7) can be integrated here as well. For example, using reflective listening to capture and reflect back client ideas about change is very valuable here and invites the client to further develop his or her ideas and plans. In doing so, the skill of gently encouraging elaboration, while not being "too far ahead" of the client's statements, is also relevant here.

Consider the following example of possible therapist responses to a client-proposed change step that either discourage ("too far ahead") or encourage client elaboration:

> CLIENT: Well, I could try to reduce my checking of the door to my apartment before I leave.
>
> THERAPIST: [too far ahead, overstating] That's a great idea! That sounds like it would certainly be a step in the right direction. When do you think you might start that?
>
> THERAPIST: [nurturing change talk and gently encouraging further elaboration] So, you're thinking that might be worth trying or playing around with. Can you say more about exactly why or how you think that would be useful?
>
> or
>
> THERAPIST: [nurturing change talk and gently encouraging further elaboration] I see. If you were to try that, how exactly would you go about that?
>
> or
>
> THERAPIST: [nurturing change talk and gently encouraging further elaboration] From what you've told me, I can imagine that would be challenging. What makes you think that that might be a good idea even though it would likely be hard?

The overly enthusiastic response assumes that the client is further ahead in his or her process of considering the action step than he or she may be, communicates pressure to change, and may be interpreted as a therapist agenda for the client to change (rather than being focused on building client arguments and plans for change). Importantly, such an overstated response runs the risk of diverting movement away from change (or counterchange talk, resistance). That is, the client is likely to respond by backing away from further elaborating change plans and/or by articulating reasons not to pursue this action (e.g., "Yeah. But it would be hard," or "I've tried that before and couldn't do it").

Enthusiastic responses to the client's early efforts can communicate pressure to change.

In contrast, undershooting in reflecting client attempts to envision change steps is far less threatening for the client, and therefore much more likely to allow the client to continue elaborating and envisioning his or her action statements (ideas and plans for change). And this is especially true when such statements are initially offered, when client commitment to such plans may be especially fragile, tenuous, and vulnerable to being easily displaced by the previously powerful status quo position. Good therapists likely have an intuitive sense to be gentle when clients begin to approach the difficult, daunting, and frightening prospect of implementing change to replace often habitual, safe, and automatic ways of being. In MI such sensitivities and skills for sustaining momentum toward change (elaborating change talk, protecting client autonomy, rolling with resistance) are made explicit.

In addition to gently encouraging elaboration of possible change steps, therapists can also help the client anticipate possible ways of addressing the obstacles and barriers to the client's plans that will likely emerge. Many of the recommendations offered in Part III of this volume, Understanding Ambivalence and Building Resolve, can be useful at this stage of action planning as well. That is, clients can be helped to articulate the arguments that the nonchange position offers to derail their efforts and then helped to examine and respond to these effectively (see especially Chapters 7 and 8). For example: "That sounds hard, and I can imagine that your anxiety will try to talk you out of doing X. What, if anything, could you say to that part of you that tries to convince you it's not worth trying?"

Conceptualizing Experiments with Change

Rather than being primarily focused on change, framing action steps as experiments whose primary goal is to gather information and whose benefit is to be tested rather than assumed can also be useful in encouraging client consideration of such activities. That is, the client may elect to try a particular action step in order to gather important information about existing beliefs/assumptions and ways of being. And there is no apriori assumption that the exercise or effort will be beneficial (in fact, it might turn out not to be). This further frees the client from pressure to change and protects client freedom of choice. For example:

> "It could be true that if you force yourself to go for a walk a few times this week and do the dishes that it won't make any difference at all in how you feel. At the same time, there's a hypothesis that you're developing that it might be useful. So, this might be a way of finding out where the truth lies. And afterward, of course, you can always stick with what you're doing now if that makes more sense in light of the new information. . . . "

Or:

"Your anxiety tells you that everyone's a critic and if you start a conversation there will be awkwardness and people will judge you and discount you. You seem to have some doubts about that, and in the absence of experience, of course, you simply don't know whether it's true or not. So, it might be worth trying something different just to find out where the truth lies. If the world is as your anxiety says it is, that would indeed be very important information to know. Right now you're just guessing, but in either case it might be important to find out so that you can figure out the best way to proceed."

This is consistent with an approach further detailed by Arkowitz (2002), who has suggested the use of the term *experiment* rather than homework. Such experiments are consistent with a spirit of discovery (rather than compliance with a therapist directive or apriori agenda for change). If the client does not engage in the activity, this is an opportunity to learn valuable information about the obstacles to change that emerge for the client. In other words, the experiment doesn't have "to work," as any outcome provides useful information. The evocative processing of such efforts to experiment with different ways of being is elaborated below.

Processing Efforts to Change

In processing the results of the client's efforts to take action toward change, the therapist can bring an attitude of curiosity to the client's experience. This promotes an atmosphere of discovery that underlies the spirit of MI. That is, when the client shows evidence of a willingness to take action, therapists have an opportunity to explore the instance as an illustration of the client's potential for change and to support his or her self-efficacy in achieving change.

Here, it is important to not assume that the client will continue with these changes (only the client can determine that) and to not immediately move in with praise or reinforcement (e.g., "That's great that you did that"); both of these reactions can communicate an attitude of compliance with the therapist's agenda for the client to change or take action. Rather, the therapist should deliberately suspend his or her own reactions or judgments in order make space for *the client* to explore, discover, and process the worth, significance, learning, or value of the experience for him- or herself. That is, the emphasis is on the client's

> *Suspend your own reactions to the client's efforts to change; let the client discover the value of the experience for himself.*

own decision making, not forcing particular desirable behavior from the therapist's perspective.

Table 9.2 presents some examples that can reflect or instantiate this spirit of curiosity and preservation of client autonomy when processing client efforts to change.

Clinical Example of Processing Change Steps

Consider the following illustration of a client whose main presenting complaint centered on obsessive "pondering" and reflection of possible future outcomes. He felt that he could not move forward in his life (e.g., taking a job, entering a university program) until he achieved a sense of certainty in the direction. As a result, he experienced a sense of paralysis in his life and continual indecisiveness, spending countless hours contemplating various options and possible outcomes. He and the therapist worked on developing an experiment that involved setting limits on obsessive pondering, limiting it to 2 hours a day, in order to gather new information about the necessity and utility of "pondering" by suspending it temporarily. In the following session the client reported that he followed through on executing the limit-setting exercise.

For contrast, let us first consider how this instance of taking an initial step toward change might be processed (and unfold) when the therapist has an allegiance to promoting change (MI-inconsistent) versus how it might be processed when the therapist has an attitude of facilitating client discovery (i.e., an MI-consistent attitude). Each of these examples is annotated to illustrate important underlying interpersonal messages with each style.

CHANGE-ORIENTED PROCESSING (MI-INCONSISTENT)

THERAPIST: Good for you for trying that. That's terrific! [reinforcement; implies conditional regard]

CLIENT: Yeah, I guess. It's a start.

THERAPIST: Well, I certainly think this is a positive step, because you haven't been able to do this before. What did you learn by doing that that you wouldn't have learned if you didn't do it? [The latter question seems evocative but is delivered in the context of a clear therapist agenda for the client to "agree" that the experiment was worthwhile.]

CLIENT: Well, I did have moments of feeling more relaxed. (*pause*) But they didn't last. [therapist allegiance to the value of the experiment risks eliciting such resistance if the client is ambivalent about its value]

TABLE 9.2. Client-Centered Ways of Responding to Efforts to Change

- "What did you like or not like about it?"
- "What did you learn, if anything, about your anxious/depressed thinking?"
- "Was it worth doing? [If yes:] Why?"
- "Would you do it again [or something similar]? Why or why not?"
- "If you continued to do this, or things like it, what do you imagine would happen? How would you feel? Good thing? Not-so-good thing?"
- "Did you learn anything that you could use to inform or help with future similar experiments or efforts you might decide on? [If yes:] What?"
- "If you were to do it again, what would you do differently, if anything?"
- "How did you get past that part of your brain that tried to talk you out of it?"
- "How did you deal with the anxiety's/depression's objections?"
- "What does doing this say about you?"

THERAPIST: Of course not. This is still very early in the process. But that's good that you did have some moments of being more relaxed. At least it's further ahead than you were before. [The therapist does not hear or "roll with" client resistance but rather seeks to defend the value of the experiment; clearly has an agenda.]

CLIENT: I guess . . . but it's hard. [continued resistance]

THERAPIST: Naturally, change is very difficult. You're going against the usual, habitual style that you're so used to. So, you can expect that it will be challenging. But with practice it should start to feel natural. [The therapist is convincing and persuading; is not letting the client have the freedom to explore the limits or possible futile aspects of the experiment.]

CLIENT: I don't know. Maybe. [continued resistance]

DISCOVERY-ORIENTED PROCESSING (MI-CONSISTENT)

THERAPIST: So, the idea behind setting these limits was to experiment with it—to find out whether doing something different would help or not. So, what are your thoughts about the results of the experiment . . . about what you've been doing? Good thing, not so good thing. [The therapist makes it clear from the beginning that he or she is interested in the client's thoughts about the value of the experiment and that the client is free to find the experiment unhelpful.]

CLIENT: Good thing mostly. [change talk]

THERAPIST: How so? Say more. [asking for elaboration]

CLIENT: Well, I am feeling more relaxed actually. I feel more "in the moment" when I'm not pondering the future. Like I'm able to "get into" stuff more. [change talk]

THERAPIST: So you can immerse yourself more fully into other pursuits. And I'm guessing that that's important for you. Am I right about that? I might not be. [reflecting change talk to encourage elaboration of it; guessing that the information gleaned from the experiment is important to the client, but again makes it clear that it is up to the client—and not the therapist—to determine this]

CLIENT: Yes. Like, my girlfriend has noticed that I'm not as distracted . . . not as much in my head. [change talk]

THERAPIST: And that makes you feel . . . [inviting elaboration]

CLIENT: . . . more normal. More able to enjoy stuff. [change talk]

THERAPIST: Anything else that's good about setting limits on the pondering? Like, I'm impressed for example that you were able to do it. It says something about you . . . that you're capable of setting limits on the obsessive thoughts . . . of fighting back. But that could just be my impression. What do you think? [affirmation; again makes it clear that this is just an observation from the therapist's own perspective and that the client is free to reject it]

CLIENT: Yeah. I'm so used to just letting them happen whenever they want to, but now I can distance myself from them a bit more. [change talk]

THERAPIST: You can exert some control over them. You don't just have to let them do or appear whenever they want. And this experiment was partly to test to see if anything bad would happen when you didn't spend all your time pondering. What's the verdict there? [reflection of change talk; encouraging further exploration of the value of the experiment]

CLIENT: Nothing bad so far. But I do worry that I'm moving forward without thinking things through enough. [Resistance emerges because the client is not 100% convinced of the value of the experiment.]

THERAPIST: I see. That maybe you're setting yourself up for a fall . . . a bad decision . . . because you're limiting the pondering. So, You're feeling more relaxed and focused, but maybe this could be dangerous in the end. And only you can judge whether the risk is worth taking. What do you think? Is this something that is worth continuing . . . it may not be? [The therapist's rolling with resistance illustrates that he or she is fully prepared to hear the client-determined limits of the experiment.]

CLIENT: I think it is, actually. I think that's the same trap that I've been falling into . . . that if I just think about things enough I can be certain and then able to relax. [When clients are free to make their own determination, they decide to err on the side of the value of the experiment; importantly, the client arrives at this conclusion free from any therapist allegiance to this conclusion.]

THERAPIST: So, it may actually work the opposite way. If I'm hearing you right, waiting until you have it all figured out hasn't really delivered what it's promised . . . hasn't led to you being relaxed or able to pursue the things that are important to you. But putting limits on that type of thinking is proving to be more helpful, at least for now, in getting to where you want to be. Is that right? [summarizing; and again inviting the client to determine the accuracy of the conclusions against his or her own experience]

Exploring the client's efforts to change in the more MI-consistent way explicitly preserves the client's autonomy and is focused on client discovery. That is, the client is free to find the experiment or step toward change unhelpful. And conducting the experiment or making efforts to change is not regarded as fulfillment of an expectation on the part of the therapist but rather as something the client has chosen and can freely evaluate for him- or herself in the context of the client's objectives, desires, and goals. In the MI-consistent approach, the therapist actively works to cultivate and maintain an "experimental" attitude, with the client as the arbiter of the utility and value of their joint efforts; and the client is free to decide to continue taking action toward change or not, depending on this assessment. The only resistance that arises in the MI-consistent segment above is the client's own internal resistance to or ambivalence about change. And this is expected and natural in the early stages of taking action toward change. The therapist then helps the client further process his or her own internal objections to change that arise in this context by rolling with this resistance.

Thus, the MI-informed approach to process action steps minimizes resistance to the therapist (that a change-oriented attitude is more likely to elicit) because the therapist is not inhabiting or taking a position that the client can disagree with or object to. That is, there is no pressure for conformity or achieving a particular outcome, only a willingness to help the client explore his or her own experience and make his or her own decisions based on that experience. Moreover, when support for autonomy is communicated by the therapist (i.e., "You can come to whatever conclusions make sense to you"), the client is much more likely to internalize the change and err on the side of articulating the benefits of the experiment or change effort (i.e., change talk). In contrast, if the therapist holds and communicates an agenda that errs on the side of change, the client is more likely to err on the side of elaborating the

When you express support for autonomy, the client is much more likely to internalize the change.

limitations or problems with the experiment in an effort to defend against the therapist's change agenda (i.e., thereby protecting his or her own freedom of choice).

Also note that the MI-consistent approach to processing steps to change in no way inhibits the therapist from mentioning possible insights, suggestions, or consequences that may be significant or important from their own perspective. In the example above, the therapist also explored important outcomes from the perspective of perceived control over obsessive thinking and whether catastrophic predictions were borne out in the client's experience. In addition, the therapist can bring in affirmations later in the exploration, for example, "I think that took a lot of courage," or "What you did is really impressive." The key is recognizing that these are your own thoughts and reactions (and may not be part of the client's experience), holding these tentatively for the client to accept or reject, and letting go of persisting with these if the suggestion or affirmation does not resonate with the client.

Bracketing an allegiance to change is not easy. This is especially the case when it seems clear that the steps the client has taken are "obviously" positive. However, subordinating your own aspirations and desires in favor of the client's continued movement toward change can be a most powerful strategy in supporting the client's own discoveries. It can also be more productive in encouraging further momentum to change.

To illustrate the importance of bracketing an allegiance to or advocacy for change when processing client action steps, consider the following example. This client suffered from depression and significant health anxiety. The client often agonized over decisions regarding future pursuits, and a central aspect of her depression and fear of dying was a concern about not having amounted to anything in her life. This client came in to the fourth session indicating substantive changes, including (1) deciding to go back to school (a major issue in previous sessions) and taking concrete steps toward this such as telling her parents and approaching them for financial support; (2) using deep breathing to focus on her anxiety instead of her usual avoidant behaviors in response to somatic symptoms; and (3) buying a journal and using it daily to become more aware of her negative thinking.

THERAPIST: Wow! It sounds like you've taken a number of significant steps.

CLIENT: I don't think so . . . maybe a little.

THERAPIST: Well, from where I sit, it sounds pretty significant, but that's just my two cents for whatever it's worth. But it's not what I think that's important—it's what *you* think that matters here. And what I hear you saying is "I've got work to do. I'm not where I want to be yet." Is that right?

CLIENT: Absolutely. Maybe I'm starting to get there, but I need to keep working at it.

Here the therapist was guessing that the client viewed her recent efforts to change as significant, but is quickly corrected by the client. The therapist was initially startled by the client's response and needed to quickly double back (roll with resistance) in favor of exploring the client's perceptions. The therapist demonstrated a willingness to let go of her own reaction to the client's efforts, takes ownership of her own response, and explicitly communicates a willingness to err on the side of favoring and exploring the client's own perceptions. Much of the session was then spent learning from and exploring the client's perceptions of the efficacy of her recent efforts, building self-efficacy, and detailing her plans for continuing change.

The therapist also *later* offered her own reflections and observations for the client to consider, for example, "I could be wrong about this, but it seems you might have some trouble taking credit where credit is due. Like, it might be scary somehow to say 'I am making progress or changing.'" This resulted in a very productive discussion of the client's self-critical style and ambivalence about relinquishing this well-practiced style (i.e., the fear of being kinder to herself and giving herself credit). Again, note here that the therapist can and should bring in their own reactions—but at the appropriate time and in a tentative manner, for the client to either accept or reject. In this case, the therapist's observation was explored only after much empathic reflection and deference to the client's agenda and experience, and it was also presented tentatively for the client to verify or deny. If, for example, this difficulty in taking credit observed by the therapist was shared earlier, such as immediately after the client's response "I don't think the steps I've taken are that significant" (e.g., with a comment like "Well, it seems that you might have trouble taking credit where credit is due"), this would communicate a lack of empathy and an unwillingness to process the client's experience and would likely be met with further resistance to the therapist's insistence on her own favored perception of events.

Bracketing Therapist-Centered Beliefs about How Change Occurs

Operating within an MI-infused framework also assumes that clients are free to (and do) change at any time. Moreover, such changes do not necessarily have to be initiated by the therapist or therapy process. In other words, if the client is dependent on the therapist's expertise (e.g., teaching specific coping skills), then one would naturally expect that clients only change after the therapist has introduced the requisite concepts and skills. A client-as-expert framework opens up other possibilities for client change that are less therapist-dependent.

As noted earlier, it is not uncommon for clients to "spontaneously" start taking action toward change when their resolve to change increases. Operating in an MI-infused manner means expecting and being alert for such client changes—in whatever form—even if they have not previously been the focus of therapy sessions. Clients can often regard these as 'small' steps. However, they can indeed be quite significant in that they reflect deviation from the usual coping style and some significant resolution of ambivalence about change (i.e., a behavioral commitment to change). These instances can also be used as a springboard for curiosity and enhancing client self-efficacy (as outlined above), and it is important for the therapist to be aware of and build on these efforts.

For example, I recall working with a therapist operating within a CBT framework who was struggling with a client and asked me to view the tape of the previous session before supervision. I was intrigued to find that the client was articulating many instances of movement toward change that the therapist did not seem to "see" (since these were not previously discussed in sessions or assigned for homework). For example, the client was highly indecisive and complained that she couldn't make even the most minor decisions. When she would go to a restaurant, she would agonize over whether to get the chicken or the fish, for example. But if she selected the chicken, she concluded that she should have ordered the fish, and vice versa. In the session, the client noted that she came across a magazine article recently in which its author stated: "You know, life is full of uncertainty and risk. The right decision is rarely clear and we just have to wade in amidst all this uncertainty, knowing that many times we'll be wrong. But that's okay. It's just life." The client said this article really got her thinking, and the next time she went to a restaurant she confidently ordered the fish—with no regrets. Then, she began to muse about what this new attitude would look like for her if she applied it more broadly. The therapist seemed to not hear the creative problem solving that the client was doing and, rather, seemed preoccupied with his own thoughts and plans (jotting down notes, looking away in reflection, etc.). Then the therapist delivered his view of the problem, which was met with resistance and generally not well received.

In supervision, when I asked the therapist to articulate his assumptions while doing CBT, he was able to identify a belief that "clients change after I introduce the methods of change" (i.e., therapist-as-expert). I asked him to view the portion of the session where the client was discussing the magazine article that she read while temporarily suspending his own beliefs (i.e., that client change occurs only after the therapist's intervention) and adopting the alternative belief that "clients do not need my permission to change." He recognized the client's self-initiated attempts at change and was quite surprised to realize that he had missed these. I reassured him that he need not worry since, when clients are in this mode, they continue to bring in other instances of active efforts to change. Consequently there would be other opportunities to notice and build on these. He subsequently worked successfully with this client to continue to hear and build on the client's self-initiated change efforts, then she used them as a springboard for discussing and integrating other similar change strategies derived from CBT (e.g., "That's really interesting and fits with what we know about developing skill at tolerating uncertainty as a way of reducing worry"). In other words, he was able to subordinate his own assumptions about how change occurs, and he found a different way of bringing in his expertise while prioritizing and seizing opportunities to prize and elaborate the client's expertise.

Helping Clients Answer Their Own Questions

Another opportunity to elicit the client's expertise prior to offering your perspective occurs when clients ask questions or ask for direction. Client questions can represent many things, and it is important to attend to the context in which they are asked. For example, at times client questions can represent genuine interest in your opinion and input; these times most often occur when the client is productively working in the action phase. At other times, questions can actually be statements reflecting skepticism about the therapy or the therapist (e.g., "How long have you been doing this?," "Have you ever seen a client like me before?," "Does CBT actually work?") In these cases, it is important to identify, explore, and roll with the resistance. For example, the therapist might say, "It sounds like you might have some important concerns about therapy. Can you say more?"

In many cases, questions or requests for direction can represent the client acting consistently with an interpersonal expectation that he or she should defer to the therapist. However, clients typically know much more than they realize. Thus, evocatively turning the question back on the client for him or her to answer (or answer first) is a useful strategy in developing self-efficacy that reflects trust in the client's inherent expertise.

Consider the following example of a client with health anxiety that occurred later in therapy:

CLIENT: There are still times when I feel that I have to check my body. I figure if I just keep busy, then that should help. What do you think?

THERAPIST: I could certainly share my opinion on that if you like, but it seems that you have some thoughts about this strategy yourself.

CLIENT: I know distraction is not very helpful. It works for a while, but then the worry just comes back. But I don't know what else to do.

THERAPIST: So, that's been your experience. And I would echo that, based on what we know about distraction from research. It can actually keep the worry going. For example, if I tell you not to think about your nose right now, how well does that work?

CLIENT: I'm thinking about it. I see.

THERAPIST: So, when you try to stop thoughts, ironically you actually make sure they stick around. But I also hear you searching for what else to do in the absence of using distraction, and maybe we can bat around some ideas there. How does that sound?

Clients typically get the message quickly that the therapist is more interested in hearing from them and in making them dig within themselves to find the information they seek. Other clients have more trouble with this, and repeated requests for direction and advise can represent an interpersonal pattern of deference that stems from doubts about being able to trust their own thoughts or experiences. Again, in these cases, an evocative approach that elicits, expects, and prioritizes client expertise is valuable.

Consider the following example of a young man presenting with recurrent major depression who repeatedly requested my advice and direction. He had a longstanding pattern of interpersonal deference and lived at home with two highly dominating parents who continually made demands on him. These issues seemed to be major contributors to his problems with depression, since he had limited self-efficacy in expressing his needs or being assertive with his parents. In fact, when using MI to build motivation in the early stage of therapy, he became aware that, in part, the depression functioned to send this interpersonal message to his family: "Leave me alone. Don't make demands on me. I need space. I need a break." Not surprisingly, then, his pattern of deference was also repeated in the therapeutic relationship, where he frequently pushed for advice and direction (i.e., he pushed for me to dominate the process).

As just one illustration of being more evocative or deferring to and eliciting the client's expertise, consider the following beginning of a later session:

THERAPIST: What would you like to put on the agenda today?

CLIENT: I don't know. Why don't you decide?

THERAPIST: You know, Sue, I've learned the hard way that what I have to say is often quite irrelevant (*laughing*). And what you have to say can be far more important. And I know it's hard to put your thoughts out there sometimes, but if you're willing I'd like to see what comes up for you. (*pause, gently*) What's on your mind?

CLIENT: (*long pause*) Actually, I was thinking about something we talked about last week. I've been thinking lately that—I am important, too.

This exchange led to a very productive discussion of the client's own needs and feelings with respect to being continually directed by others. Importantly, had I accepted his invitation to set the agenda, I would have further undermined his autonomy and self-efficacy. Thus, an attitude of seeking to actively elicit and prioritize client expertise (especially when the client feels he or she doesn't have the requisite expertise) can be particularly helpful and needed for some clients.

SUMMARY AND CONCLUSION

MI therapists believe that clients have inherent but undiscovered expertise and wisdom regarding change. At the action stage, this wisdom includes client knowledge and expertise about how to resolve problems and develop solutions to accomplish the changes they seek. When supporting clients in developing a vision and plan for possible steps to achieve change, therapists working within the MI spirit seek to systematically and preferentially tap into these existing and inherent ideas, thoughts, and preferences of the client about how best to change. Working from an MI perspective at this stage also means supporting and guiding clients in further elaborating and developing their ideas. Here, therapists can sensitively seek to nurture the fuller elaboration and exploration of client ideas and plans for change by responding in a way that reduces the risk of resistance and encourages further movement toward change. Moreover, infusing MI into therapeutic work at this stage also means being careful to protect client autonomy with respect to decisions about how to change and to avoid pressuring clients to persist with change.

In seeking to evoke and build on client expertise, and supporting and guiding clients to envision steps to change, the MI therapist not only helps the client develop greater commitment to and confidence in taking action to change but also ultimately facilitates greater client self-determination and trust in his or her own inherent resources (i.e., increases his or her self-efficacy). Throughout this process, the therapist also contributes valuable and integral resources/expertise in helping clients develop and envision possibilities for achieving change and in implementing their efforts to change. How MI can inform the integration of such therapist expertise is further considered in the next chapter.

10

❦

Sharing Your Expertise

INTEGRATING DIRECTIVE
AND SUPPORTIVE APPROACHES

As we have seen in the preceding chapter, the MI therapist continually seeks to evoke the client's ideas, perspectives, preferences, and proposed solutions with respect to change. Operating from this MI spirit means evoking client thoughts and ideas prior to contributing your own. The therapist works to avoid imposing his or her own ideas and preferred methods about how change should be accomplished, in order to avoid coercing clients to conform to his or her own agenda.

What, then, is the role of therapist expertise? At a superficial glance, in this more supportive way of working it can seem that there is less of a role for the therapist—who simply defers to the client's wisdom and gets out of the way so clients can heal themselves. But recall (see Chapter 2 on the MI spirit) that from an MI perspective much of the therapist's expertise resides in the important task of facilitating the process of therapy and getting clients actively engaged in this process. Stated differently, while the client is the expert on the content, the therapist is an invaluable expert on the process, in creating the conditions that allow client expertise to be realized and solutions to emerge.[1]

But what about the therapist's considerable expertise and knowledge? This might include (but not be limited to):

---

[1] Similarly, process–experiential therapies draw a distinction between being process-directive and content-directive (e.g., Greenberg et al., 1993).

- Solutions to the pernicious problems of anxiety and related problems, such as depression.
- A wealth of expertise regarding the factors maintaining such problems.
- Knowledge of various effective (and ineffective) approaches to resolving and helping clients free themselves from these highly aversive affective states.
- Direct experience with clients that can be offered as feedback on clients' interpersonal styles and habitual ways of relating.
- Specific coping skills that are often useful to those with anxiety and related problems.
- Knowledge of the research on the characteristics of these disorders and the actions stemming from this knowledge that are helpful to sufferers in overcoming these disabling conditions.

Should this wealth of knowledge be abandoned in the service of helping clients "heal themselves"? Quite the contrary—such expertise, input, and feedback can be and often are extremely useful and indeed integral in guiding clients to realize their goals for change. There is no question about their value. In fact, not contributing such input and guidance could be experienced (accurately) as withholding to clients. As Rogers (1951) notes:

> In the first place, some counsellors have supposed that the counsellor's role in carrying on nondirective counselling was merely to be passive and to adopt a laissez faire policy. He tries to "stay out of the client's way." This misconception of the approach has led to considerable failure in counselling—and for good reasons. The passivity and seeming lack of interest or involvement is experienced by the client as a rejection, since indifference is in no real way the same as acceptance. In the second place, a laissez faire attitude does not in any way indicate to the client that he is regarded as a person of worth. (p. 27)

Yet, effectively integrating more and less directive approaches can be challenging. For the therapist used to being successful with a more directive style, a more supportive approach can be difficult to adopt and work with. For years, I had a critic on my shoulder (that still reemerges every now and again) that would attack me when I went into a supportive mode. It would say something like, "Don't just listen. Do something!" Interestingly, I learned that client-centered therapists have the opposite dilemma, experiencing an inner critic whenever they consider being more directive (Elliott, personal communication) that might say something like "Don't do anything—just listen." In attempting to integrate my directive with my less directive self, I would often experience the worst of both worlds, alternating between both critics (talk about being stuck!). Thus, being both directive and supportive, and moving seamlessly between these two ways of being, can be a daunting task.

Therapist expertise can come in many forms, including (but not limited to) information or psychoeducation, a suggestion or advice on how to accomplish the desired change, teaching a skill, a reaction or piece of feedback, or an interpretation. Whatever the form, such valuable guidance and additions to client efforts to change can be introduced and processed in a way that enhances the probability of client engagement with these therapist offerings. Of particular importance is protecting and reinforcing client autonomy and freedom of choice, since such inputs emerge from your own perspective, not the client's, and therefore carry a higher risk of client resistance or opposition. Also, explicit monitoring of client receptivity and his or her level of engagement with such offerings is important. These points are further elaborated and illustrated below.

MAKING SUGGESTIONS
WHILE PRESERVING CLIENT AUTONOMY

Any therapist idea, feedback, or suggestion by definition comes from a nonjoined frame of reference (versus the joined frame of reference employed in empathic reflection) and therefore carries a much higher risk of being met with resistance (i.e., opposition to the therapist, arguments against change). To elaborate, when listening empathically you are operating from a joined perspective (e.g., "If I hear you right, you are saying . . . ") or even speaking *as if* you are the client (e.g., "Others will reject me," "I can't stand it"). As Rogers (1975) outlined, when being empathic you are attempting to see and sense the world as the client senses it—to temporarily inhabit his or her frame of reference. In a sense, it as if one person—the client—is speaking. In this context, resistance to the therapist is virtually nonexistent since there is no one to resist or oppose. However, your own perspective, ideas, reactions, suggestions, thoughts, and the like (e.g., "I think . . . ," "Why don't you . . . ," "What about . . . ," "I see it this way . . . ") are separate from this. As I have been arguing, these are very valuable to communicate and bring forward for the client to consider. Using the MI spirit to inform this process involves sensitivity to how such inputs are delivered, particularly, to issues of client autonomy. The therapist significantly reduces the risk of resistance and increases the probability of engagement by carefully communicating (both implicitly and explicitly) recognition that the client is totally free to accept, adapt, or reject the suggestion or feedback as he or she sees fit.

Thus, contributing your perspective by using the MI spirit means:

- Recognizing it is *your* perspective and not currently the client's.
- "Holding it lightly" (tentatively) with an attitude of "information for the client to possibly consider if he or she chooses to do so."

> Contributing a suggestion in the MI spirit means being prepared to drop it if the client rejects it

- Being prepared to back off from your suggestion, idea, or position if the client rejects it or is not prepared to engage with it (i.e., shows resistance).

Below I outline several major areas, in working with clients with anxiety and related problems, where therapist input and suggestions (external expertise) are often very helpful in advancing client thinking, solutions, and movement toward change. In particular, I consider how to integrate the MI spirit of preserving autonomy into (1) helping clients question their assumptions or underlying beliefs through Socratic questioning, (2) providing feedback and psychoeducation, and (3) guiding the application of specific skills or coping methods. These examples are used to illustrate how one can contribute therapist expertise while explicitly safeguarding client autonomy and freedom of choice. These principles may apply to any time the therapist offers his or her own expertise, not just to these illustrations.

Socratic Questioning, Motivational Interviewing Style

A major task of treatment for those wrestling with anxiety and related problems such as depression involves helping clients become aware of and critically examine their existing assumptions or underlying beliefs that perpetuate anxiety or depression. That is, clients need to be helped to explore and critically evaluate their existing beliefs that lead to the negative affect they experience as well as to develop and elaborate healthier and more adaptive alternative perspectives. In addition to encouraging the use of a joined perspective to accomplish this task (i.e., empathic listening), there are many opportunities to further the development of alternative, less anxiety-arousing, perspectives by contributing your thoughts and suggestions (nonjoined perspective) for the client to consider. In CBT, this is referred to as Socratic questioning, or the process of prompting clients to critically question the existing assumptions and belief systems perpetuating the problems they are seeking relief from. Drawing on both perspectives—the client's and your own—to deconstruct and evaluate the client's existing set of assumptions promotes a collaborative atmosphere in which both parties bring expertise to this important task.

When done with the MI spirit, this means often explicitly communicating freedom of choice. Importantly, questions and suggestions about alternative perspectives that are offered by the therapist are not intended to convince the client of the truth or to correct errant ways of thinking. Rather, they are introduced as possibilities for the client to consider and explore if he or she chooses to do so. That is, based on MI principles, engaging in Socratic questioning is not an exercise in persuasion but rather a form of communication that reflects your active willingness and effort to brainstorm in concert with the client about various possibilities to put on the table for consideration (i.e., a food for thought)—with the client as the sole arbiter of whether the possibilities are retained and further explored or, instead, rejected. Encouraging such self-confrontation in this way involves implicitly (in your own attitude—reminding yourself that it is the client who gets to decide) and

> *When Socratic questioning is done in the MI spirit, the client is generally more receptive to suggestions.*

explicitly (articulating and reinforcing client control and freedom of choice) preserving client autonomy. When Socratic questioning is done in this spirit, it can increase the probability of client receptivity to therapist suggestions and contributions to this process.

Table 10.1 presents some examples of helping clients to reevaluate their existing assumptions that instantiate the MI spirit of preserving autonomy. When presenting the issues in this way, you are explicitly communicating a respect for the client's autonomy and a recognition of his or her authority in making choices. That is, statements such as these make it clear that the client does not have to accept that there is an alternative perspective or choose to explore this possibility in that moment. Here, you are merely asking him or her to consider the possibility and the client is free to accept this invitation or not. You are also affirming the client's right to continue with the existing thinking style (i.e., he or she doesn't have to change). In other words, the therapist lets go of the idea that the client should change his or her thinking and leaves this up to the client to decide. Ironically, when the client's freedom to choose is explicitly and implicitly preserved in the therapist's communication, it makes it much more likely that the client will consider the idea that there might be a different way of thinking (resulting in a reduced probability of resistance). Greenberger and Padesky's (1995) style of examining evidence for and against a belief also has this spirit of exploration in the service of client decision making and implicitly communicates that the client is free to decide.

Notice that this way of framing therapist inputs and suggestions

TABLE 10.1. Examples of Socratic Questions That Preserve Client Autonomy

- "It could be true that you need to be perfect in order for others to want to spend time with you. What do you think? True? Not true?"
- "Your anxiety says that if you worry you can prevent bad things from happening. Is there a part of you that disagrees with that. There may not be."
- "I'm not sure about this and it could be wrong, but I wonder if there is another way of thinking about this situation? For example, could it be possible that . . . ?"
- "See what you think about this. It may not fit at all, but I wonder if another way of looking at this is. . . . "
- "What occurred to me as you were talking was . . . but that might be a stretch—it might not fit for you."
- *Client*: If people really knew me they wouldn't like me. I'm boring.
  Therapist: Only you can know for sure if that's true—and it might be. I wonder if it might be equally true that you have *moments* of being boring—like we all do—but that doesn't mean you are boring person. But I could be way off on that. What do you think?
- "There's this idea that other people think you're stupid. If you were to take issue with that—and you don't have to—what, if anything, could you say to that?"
- If the client has achieved some awareness of his or her values or authentic self: "So, the insecure voice says, 'No one likes you, and they never will.' What does George [the client's name] think of that? [or "What do *you* think of that?"] True? Not true?"

---

draws on the use of tentativeness, which is more commonly considered and discussed in the context of empathic listening (e.g., "Do I have that right?," "If I hear you right, you are saying . . . ," "I'm not sure about this, but I think I hear . . . Would that be true?"). Here, this concept has been extrapolated to any therapist input and arguably is especially important when contributing suggestions and direction from the therapist's own frame of reference. For example, in offering suggestions about alternative perspectives in the context of Socratic questioning, there is potentially a higher risk of becoming attached to one's own inputs (preferred perspectives, efforts to be helpful, etc.). Thus, explicit recognition that this is your own perspective (being especially careful to communicate that you are not wedded to these ideas), and working hard to nurture and protect your client's freedom of choice (to reject your perspective) at these times are key elements.

Accordingly, I find that it's very important to not only implicitly hold this attitude but also *explicitly* communicate that the client is "free to decide" when using Socratic questioning. This is because it can be very easy to lose this spirit and fall into pushing for change or pressuring the client to adopt the healthier perspective. Thus, by being judiciously explicit about communicating client autonomy and self-determination, you not only convey to the client that he or she is free to decide which perspective to endorse but also remind yourself of the truth—namely, that only the client can know what is best! Becoming too attached to your suggestions (no matter how clever and incisive they may be) communicates to the client that he or she should "think like you think," thereby undermining clients' critical task of exploring and evaluating their existing ways of being for themselves.

Clients can be exquisitely sensitive to attempts to undermine their autonomy and can be highly attuned to signs that the therapist is pushing for change (directly or indirectly) or "has an agenda" for the "right way" to think. Importantly, becoming attached to your perspective and inputs typically makes it less rather than more likely that they will be well received. Pushing the development of an alternative perspective also places clients in the uncomfortable position of having to risk hurting or rejecting you (since it is clear that you are attached to your viewpoint or your need to be helpful) in order to assert their autonomy. Clients may then acquiesce—but solely in order to avoid this risk, preserve your involvement, and safeguard the therapeutic alliance. Thus, it needs to be very clear in the therapist's communications (both verbally and nonverbally) that clients are free to "go their own way" even if that means disagreeing with or going against what the therapist is suggesting.

Clinical Examples

The two examples below illustrate this use of Socratic questioning in the spirit of safeguarding client autonomy and freedom of choice. Note here that the therapist interpolates the use of Socratic questioning in an MI style, with empathic reflection to elaborate the client's responses (i.e., the therapist moves fluidly between joined and nonjoined frames of reference).

EXAMPLE 1

CLIENT: My colleagues didn't include me in that edited book or even cite my work.

THERAPIST: And what does the insecure part of you say . . . make of that? [asking for the meaning of the event]

CLIENT: I'm not really important . . . my work doesn't matter.

THERAPIST: And you worry that it never will matter. They think you're incompetent and that will never change. [empathic reflection to further guess at meaning]

CLIENT: Exactly. Like I haven't produced anything of value and never will.

THERAPIST: So, that's what the insecure voice says. Is there another part of you that might disagree? Like, how certain are you, for example, that they were deliberately excluding you because they think you're incompetent? That's a possibility of course, and you would know better than I, but I wonder if there might be other explanations that might be true too. Maybe not. What are your thoughts? [Socratic questioning in an MI style]

CLIENT: I actually know this person, and I'm pretty sure they don't regard me as incompetent. In fact, they like my work. I think they probably didn't ask me to be part of the book because they weren't aware of my previous work in that area since it's not the major thing I'm known for.

THERAPIST: So, it might be an understandable oversight rather than a message that they're sending that they see you as incompetent. [empathic reflection to encourage elaboration]

CLIENT: Actually, I think if I send my work in this area to the editors, they will be happy to see it and to be made aware of it.

THERAPIST: And what about the idea that you'll never produce anything of value? It sounds like that might already be kind of untrue from what you're saying, but only you can know. How accurate would you say that prediction is? Is there room for doubt on that or no? [Socratic questioning in an MI style]

CLIENT: Well, I'm still very early in my career. It's true that I haven't produced my most significant work yet.

THERAPIST: So, that's just the truth, but that doesn't mean you're destined to fail. Is that right? [empathic reflection to encourage elaboration]

CLIENT: Yes. In fact, if I look at it, I've been highly successful relative to my colleagues at the same level.

THERAPIST: And what if it really is true that they excluded you deliberately . . . because it might be. What, if anything, could you say about that? [Socratic questioning in an MI style]

CLIENT: Well, I highly doubt it, but if it were true, that would be unfortunate for them to totally discount me like that.

EXAMPLE 2

THERAPIST: Sometimes when other people are critical of others, it can say more about them than the person they're criticizing. Does that fit for you at all? It might not. [Socratic questioning in an MI style]

CLIENT: That's true.

THERAPIST: You seem to agree. If you're willing, can you say more?

CLIENT: Like, it could just be a reflection of their insecurities. Their need to be critical.

THERAPIST: Rather than being a reflection on you. [empathic reflection]

CLIENT: Yeah.

THERAPIST: And, if I'm hearing you right, it seems that it might be important for you to not buy into that. Like it might be important to screen criticism by where it's coming from—rather than considering it all to be equally important. Would that be true? I might be off on that, though. [empathic reflection and Socratic questioning, MI style]

CLIENT: Yes. Like, right now I just think anything negative anyone has to say about me is true.

THERAPIST: And it might not be. [empathic reflection]

CLIENT: Right. In fact, most of the time I think it's not valid.

THERAPIST: So, there are times, even a lot of them, when criticism is not valid. Assuming that all criticism is valid might be the way to go, and only you can know if it's helpful or necessary to make that kind of assumption. What do you think? [empathic reflection and Socratic questioning in an MI style]

Providing Psychoeducation and Feedback

Another common and helpful place for therapist external expertise and input is in offering psychoeducation and feedback to clients. Such inputs can be extremely valuable and welcomed by clients. These inputs could include, for example, a rationale for a particular approach to the problem, observations about the client that the therapist makes, a suggestion for a between-session activity, or particular information to help clients normalize, understand, and reconceptualize their experience, among others.

Miller and Rollnick (2002) describe the technique of *elicit–provide–elicit* when giving feedback, which is intended to communicate this "food for thought" attitude when bringing in material from an external perspective. In particular, when giving information, the therapist first asks the client's permission, then delivers the feedback, and then explicitly elicits the client's reaction to what has been offered in order to help him or her process it, make sense of it, determine whether it fits, and further integrate it if the client chooses. The critical issue in this approach is not in the technique

itself but in what it communicates
to the client, namely, recognition
that the client is the sole authority
on whether to accept the information. Again, such explicit recognition
and nurturing of client autonomy

> *"Elicit–provide–elicit"
> recognizes the client as the
> authority on whether to accept
> therapist suggestions.*

increases the probability of client receptivity to the therapist suggestion/
input.

The elicit–provide–elicit method is illustrated in the following three
clinical vignettes. They have been selected to illustrate how this method can
be used at several common junctures in working with clients with anxiety
and related problems of depression. Respectively, the examples illustrate
the introduction of a between-session activity, offering assessment feedback, and offering feedback during the course of therapy.

EXAMPLE 1: INTRODUCING A BETWEEN-SESSION ACTIVITY

THERAPIST: Can I leave you with a question to consider over the next
week? [asking permission]

CLIENT: Sure.

THERAPIST: One of the things that is emerging for you is this sense
that I have to prove myself to people a lot. I wonder if it would
be helpful to watch yourself this week, and even write down if
you like, how this works itself out in your daily life—observing
yourself with an eye to finding out specifically how this need to
prove yourself pushes you around or has you acting. This might
help us to get a better idea of how, and the degree to which,
this operates and to come up with some specific examples that
we might consider together at our next meeting. [offering the
suggestion] Does that make sense or sound like something that
would be useful at all? It might not be. [evoking client reac-
tion]

CLIENT: Yes. I can see how that might help.

THERAPIST: Can you say more about what you're thinking?

CLIENT: Well, I probably do it all the time, and without thinking. It
might help me to get a better sense of when I do it—like, with
specific people or at certain times.

Here, the therapist makes it clear that the client is free to reject the
suggestion. Moreover, the therapist is also open to the client's using the

idea as a springboard to creatively carve out better ways of proceeding with that idea or an alternative idea. Alternatively, of course, rather than using the elicit–provide–elicit method, the therapist could simply inquire "What, if anything, might make sense to do between now and the next time we meet?," which is evocative while also preserving client autonomy.

EXAMPLE 2: OFFERING FEEDBACK IN AN ASSESSMENT[2]

During an initial assessment interview (which was a diagnostic interview) with a client with severe social anxiety, it became clear that she also had a drinking problem. She was experiencing blackouts, memory loss, missing work, and had frequent conflicts with others concerned about her drinking. She clearly stated, however, that she did not believe she had a drinking problem. At the end of the interview, after offering her feedback on anxiety and related problems, I as well asked her if it was okay to give her some feedback about her drinking [asking permission]. Since she looked quite reticent about this, I reinforced that she was perfectly free to say "No" to hearing the feedback. Also I noted that, if she did decide to agree, I was merely taking the opportunity to provide her with some information relevant to the parts of the interview that she had just completed that were about drinking. I reinforced that only she could know whether the information was useful to her or not, and that she was free to discard it or think further about it, as she saw fit. With this reassurance, she agreed to hear the feedback.

I then said:

"I hear very clearly that you don't have a drinking problem and your drinking may be an issue for others but it is not a concern for you. Again, just by way of information—and you can take this for whatever it is worth—other people that do have problems with drinking tend to experience many of the same things that you have indicated— such as trouble with memory, blackouts, problems at work, and the like. Only you can know whether this is a problem for you, and no one else—no matter how expert they may claim to be—can tell you that you have a problem when you don't see it that way. If you do decide someday that it is a problem or that it becomes a problem for you, I'd be happy to talk about options for what you can do." [providing the information]

---

[2] Finn and Tonsager (1997) also outline a model that illustrates and elaborates a more exploratory client-centered approach to the process of assessment.

I then asked her, "What, if anything, do you make of that?" (eliciting the client's response). She was quite silent (reflective) for a while and eventually responded that it definitely gave her some things to think about. We proceeded on to other issues and then wrapped up the interview. To my great surprise, on her way out the door, she turned to me and said, "You know, I think I might have a drinking problem." We then proceeded to make a follow-up appointment to explore this further, build her resolve for taking action to manage her drinking, and discuss possible treatment options. Of course, giving feedback isn't always this well received (after all, we reserve our very best examples of a method for books like this). However, the probability of a client's further consideration of therapist feedback, information, and input can be significantly enhanced by judicious efforts and intentions to reinforce client autonomy; and this is probably especially needed when the feedback is highly discrepant with the client's current position or viewpoint.

EXAMPLE 3: OFFERING FEEDBACK/OBSERVATIONS DURING THE COURSE OF THERAPY

Many times during the course of therapy therapists make observations based on what they consider particularly important, such as identifying defenses against experience (e.g., "I notice that you are laughing even though what you are talking about is not funny" or "You tend change the subject whenever we talk about something that seems to touch you") or habitual patterns of responding (e.g., "When you start to cry, you feel a need to apologize—I wonder where that comes from" or "You seem to be very concerned about my impression of you—I wonder what that's about").

In the illustration below, I shared an observation that struck me as important in the course of working to help a client with recurrent depression develop greater self-compassion. I believe that self-criticism, hostility, and punishment of the self (even hatred) are very toxic—to both the client and the process of therapy. That is, they can interrupt or derail productive client exploration since the client then just focuses on berating him- or herself and ceases the process of discovery (e.g., "You see how stupid I am," "I'm such an idiot"). Thus, I like to call attention to instances of such self-hostility when they occur (e.g., "Wow, you really whip yourself!," "You can be very nasty toward yourself") in order to draw client attention to them and ultimately to pave the way for greater self-compassion. Preservation of autonomy (recognition that this emerges from the therapist's perspective and freedom to reject the observation) can be communicated implicitly and explicitly in doing so. For example,

CLIENT: That's interesting hearing you say that about being kinder to myself. I tried journaling once. I wrote down good things to remind myself of. One thing I remember that I wrote was "patience." (*pause*) But then I threw it away because it didn't last; I just slip back into that frenzied mindset anyway.

THERAPIST: (*smiling*) I find it fascinating to watch you. From where I sit, it's amazing to me to see how quickly that other voice steps in and takes charge—"You know, I tried being patient once, and it didn't work. Screw patience. Patience is overrated!"

CLIENT: (*Laughs.*)

THERAPIST: I don't know about this, but I wonder if that in itself could be an exercise in being patient. What do you think?

CLIENT: It's true. I'm not sure if I can buy the "being kinder" thing yet. But I think what I can do is be more aware of that voice and how it jumps in and takes over.

THERAPIST: Can you say more?

Interestingly, even though my suggestion (that emerged from my observation) was too far ahead of where the client was, because I consciously recognized her autonomy she ended up taking a piece of it that did resonate with her. Contrast this with more directive (less autonomy-sensitive) ways of wording suggestions, such as "What you need to do is . . . ," "I recommend that . . . ," or "What I want you to do is . . . " Such words emerge from a very different spirit, one that seeks to persuade or influence the client to the therapist's way of thinking. Thus, again it is not so much the particular observation or piece of feedback that can be critical in moving the client forward but rather the manner in which such observations are held by the therapist (through his or her attitude or spirit) and consequently delivered.

Teaching and Guiding the Application of Anxiety Reduction Methods

Another place where explicit therapist direction and expertise can be very useful is in teaching particular coping skills. Here, again, continued therapist attentiveness to preserving client autonomy and to client engagement and receptivity to such instruction is valuable. Consider the example of a client with performance anxiety, panic, and chronic perfectionism who presented to an early treatment session in a frantic state of very high anxiety. This was triggered by having made an error at work, which in turn created strong feelings of self-recrimination, rumination, and destructive urges to quit her job (e.g., "This just proves that I can't do this job. I'm not smart enough. I don't belong there") in order to escape the anxiety.

I viewed this as an opportunity both to help the client learn how to better soothe and calm herself and to illustrate and experiment with possible ways of doing so. I suggested to her that, although quitting her job might be the best thing to do in the end, major decisions such as that were typically best made when not in a highly anxious state (I also offered psychoeducation about the impact of anxiety on cognitive processing). Specifically, I observed: "You're not the greatest self-soother—and, given your history, that makes sense. I wonder if it might be worthwhile to take a few minutes to work on turning the threat switch off. Would that make sense?" [asking permission].

The client accepted this rationale and was agreeable to this way of proceeding. We then spent several minutes doing a deep breathing exercise (after which she was visibly more relaxed and less frantic). We then proceeded to work together on brainstorming a list of other possible self-soothing activities that she could use in response to anxiety by considering "What someone who is infinitely compassionate and understanding would say to her." Again, this process of brainstorming is more effective when the therapist explicitly reassures the client that he or she is free from the pressure to act on the suggestions (e.g., "You don't have to act on or use these suggestions, but let's just brainstorm what the possibilities might be for calming yourself, hypothetically. Then later you can decide which ones, if any, fit for you or make sense to experiment with"). The client then identified a range of possibilities for self-soothing, including exercising, not skipping meals, hope statements (e.g., "This too shall pass—it always does"), reminders of mood-congruent thinking ("This is just what my mind conjures up when I feel anxious"), and lowering rather than raising expectations when distressed. Thus, even in situations where the therapist takes a more explicitly directive role in teaching clients particular coping skills, continuing attentiveness to the issues of client autonomy, receptivity, and engagement is warranted.

ASSESSING CLIENT RECEPTIVITY
TO YOUR SUGGESTIONS/INPUTS

Extending the MI spirit into the entire course of therapy means that the therapist is continually and explicitly monitoring client engagement. And this is arguably especially important when offering your perspective/suggestions, given the heightened risk of resistance to the therapist at these times. Here, the therapist is constantly asking him- or herself, "Where is the client going?" for example, "Are they moving toward accepting the suggestion that I just made, or are they declining the invitation /not ready for that/going somewhere else?" This monitoring can be done both by observations (e.g., see Chapter 3) and by directly asking the client for his or her response. For example, you might ask: "Does that make sense?," "How do you hear that?," or "Is that something that might be useful to you?" In short, the issue is not being directive per se but rather ensuring that the client remains engaged.

In assessing client response to their inputs, therapists remain attentive and alert for signs of disengagement. Resistance nearly always emerges, especially during the early stages of exploring and developing alternative ways of thinking, acting, and being. It is also important to avoid assuming that the client will fully adopt an alternative viewpoint or way of being because he or she has one or two moments of clarity, affinity for, or allegiance to it. Habitual ways of being are incredibly resistant to change, even when clients are beginning to consider and take action to change them. And sometimes (even often), although we can take care to present things tentatively and in a manner supporting client autonomy, clients will still reject this input, eventually deciding it doesn't fit or is in some way unacceptable. Thus, being continually prepared to roll with this resistance is a key clinical skill in ensuring the client's continued engagement in the therapy process.

Consider the following example of client resistance in response to a therapist attempt to offer an affirmation,

THERAPIST: This is just my opinion, of course—and you can take it for whatever it's worth—but I see you as a very strong woman, someone who is a survivor. [affirmation]

CLIENT: I wish I saw it that way.

THERAPIST: I want to see myself that way, but right now I don't. There's an important part of me that says that that's not right. Can you say more about that? What keeps you from seeing it that way? [rolling with resistance]

Resistance is not cause for concern (unless, of course, it is sustained and unremitting). It often simply communicates that what we are offering is too far ahead of where the client is—how they see themselves and what they need currently. It is not a sign that the therapist is wrong, unhelpful, or misguided. Rather, it's mostly a question of timing. And it offers an opportunity for further exploration. Thus, in practice that is informed by MI, the therapist is always prepared to reframe and roll with resistance to change (see Chapter 6; the use of this critical skill when working in the action phase is further discussed in Chapter 12). In short, the therapist instantiating the MI spirit genuinely accepts the client's freedom (and wisdom) in rejecting his or her inputs and, moreover, resists trying

Client resistance is not a sign that the therapist is unhelpful or misguided.

to convince or persuade the client of the value of the inputs and suggestions when it is clear that the client is unwilling to accept them.

SUMMARY

Therapist expertise comes in many forms, including (but not limited to) effective ways of approaching problems such as anxiety and depression; observations and feedback about a client; information and psychoeducation to advance understanding of anxiety and related problems; and knowledge of particular effective coping skills in alleviating and soothing such noxious feeling states. While client-centered and supportive approaches emphasize evoking client expertise/knowledge and solutions that arise from a joined (empathic) understanding, it is inaccurate to assume that there is no role for therapist expertise that emerges from an external nonjoined perspective. In fact, integrating such therapist expertise can be invaluable and essential in guiding clients to realizing their goals for change.

Infusing MI into treatment with clients in the action stage can inform when and how to introduce therapist expertise. The therapist informed by MI is particularly attentive to protecting and preserving client autonomy and systematically monitoring receptivity/response to his or her offerings. Therapists can take preemptive steps to reduce the risk of resistance when contributing ideas from their own external frame of reference and should explicitly monitor the impact of such offerings on client engagement and disengagement. Sensitivity to these matters is particularly important since there is arguably a higher risk of client resistance (and therapist attachment) to inputs that emerge from the therapist's own knowledge and expertise. Importantly, these are not tricks or techniques that one uses to get the client to "go along" with the therapist's views on the right way to proceed. Rather, the sensitivities and skills described in this chapter emerge most effectively from centering oneself in, or operating foundationally from, the gentle, respectful, noncoercive attitude that underlies MI when properly conducted. It can be particularly important to consistently remind yourself of these principles—that is, to cultivate and nurture this attitude—when bringing in your own expertise (i.e., when being more directive), given the inherent risk of becoming too attached to our own ideas in your genuine efforts to be helpful.

11

♋

Listening Reflectively

As we have seen, when clients become interested in developing specific strategies for achieving change, the therapist then shifts to a more action-oriented mode, helping the client develop and implement change plans, offering expertise on helpful strategies for problem resolution, and teaching coping skills, psychoeducation, and the like. At these times, therapists tend to rely more on doing, teaching, or directing than on exercising skills like empathic listening. That is, while supportive skills such as empathic listening are clearly needed to build client resolve for change, envisioning a primary role for this core MI skill during the action phase of therapy is more difficult. During this phase, clients are in a "doing" mode and more receptive to and welcoming of therapist direction. In fact, therapy with a highly motivated client may proceed quite smoothly with a modest level of empathy but not require significant reliance on this skill, relative to others.

In this chapter, however, I argue for the continued judicious use and integration of the MI skill of empathic listening during the action phase of therapy. Empathy is a foundational skill in MI, but its use does not have to be restricted to managing motivational impasses or fostering the therapeutic alliance in order to gain engagement with specific recommendations for change. I argue for a view of empathic listening as an active intervention that accomplishes important and common objectives in the treatment of those suffering from anxiety and depression.

Empathy promotes increased client self-awareness, facilitates self-confrontation, and enhances access, exposure to, and acceptance of unwanted and avoided experiences (i.e., negative affect). Moreover, therapist empathic listening also promotes client self-acceptance. That is, empathy is a major vehicle through which the underlying attitudes of MI are communicated. Such experiences of being regarded by another in this accepting and nonjudgmental manner can serve as a catalyst for greater client self-regard and self-acceptance. And such experiences are especially important for clients with anxiety and depression, who suffer from chronically low self-regard and self-criticism.

EMPATHIC LISTENING TO ENCOURAGE SELF-CONFRONTATION AND EXPERIENTIAL AWARENESS

Consider the following excerpts from client-centered and process experiential approaches of some of the major functions of empathic listening:

- Empathic responses help clients to deconstruct and freely examine and reevaluate their worldviews, including their experiences, histories, assumptions, values, needs, and behaviors. As clients try to articulate and symbolize their experience, it becomes clearer and better defined; and as therapists struggle to understand and apprehend their clients' realities, they help to uncover the clients' assumptions, leaving these open to questioning and reevaluation by the client (Watson, 2001; Watson et al., 1998).
- A primary aim of empathic responding is to validate clients' perceptions and create conditions of safety and lowered threat, to allow for the formulation of new views of the self and the reorganization of self-structures (Rogers, 1975; Bozarth, 1990).
- Empathic exploration focuses clients' attention on specific aspects of their experience, especially their feelings, aspirations, and assumptions. This enables clients to reflect on their assumptions and the aspects of their experience that might be contributing to their current view, which in turn enables them to reexamine their perspectives and assumptions before determining how they wish to act (Greenberg et al., 1993).

The convergence of this deconstructive function of empathy with the objectives of many action-oriented approaches to the treatment of anxiety and related problems like depression is striking. Specifically, empathy helps clients understand and reevaluate their set of assumptions and ways of behaving. In CBT, for example, empathic listening is not generally considered a major mechanism in itself for promoting change; rather, its importance is thought to lie in maintaining the therapeutic alliance and gaining cooperation for the necessary subsequent tasks of evaluating existing assumptions and beliefs and experimenting with new ways of being. An expanded view of the role of empathic reflection for accomplishing such important objectives may be possible.

That is, like Socratic questioning, for example, empathic listening might be understood as an important vehicle or tool in *directly* facilitating clients' consideration of alternative views and responses. That is, through the process of hearing themselves more clearly and deeply and articulating their assumptions, values and objectives, the client begins to gain some distance and evaluate these perspectives and assumptions anew. In other words, empathy can play a significant role in accomplishing the important tasks of increasing self-awareness and encouraging self-confrontation (i.e., the reevaluation of underlying assumptions and ways of being).

REVISITING THE LEADING EDGE

As noted when discussing the skillful and gentle style needed to elaborate change talk (see Chapter 7), good empathic reflection involves going beyond (but not too far beyond) what the client has said. It adds nuances of meaning or experience that have not yet been stated but are clearly implicit in the client's statements. This is referred to as attempting to capture the "leading edge" (Martin, 1999). Empathy at its most highly developed level brings knowledge that is at the periphery into focus (Beech & Brazier, 1995). Rogers (1975) described the process as "temporarily living in [the client's] life, moving about in it delicately [and] sensing meanings of which he or she is scarcely aware" (p. 1833).

Empathy enables you to more fully understand and deconstruct clients' dominant views of themselves, others, and the world by bringing that which has been marginalized and silenced to center stage. In the service of this, the therapist strives to be neither behind the client (e.g., simply parroting or restating) nor too far ahead of the client (e.g., making reflections that the client is not likely to accept since they are too far outside of his or her immediate awareness), since neither of these will facilitate movement in the client's developing understanding or awareness. Rather, the therapist strives to capture the implicit

Empathy enables understanding of a client's hidden views of himor herself.

meanings that are just outside of the client's awareness but are nonetheless contained within it (Sachse & Elliott, 2001).

This process involves guessing at meanings, assumptions, or aspects of experience that the client is scarcely aware of. This is an area in which I have found my training in cognitive therapy to be invaluable. Such training helps therapists hone their skill at recognizing that there are underlying beliefs and assumptions in clients' more surface statements; it also helps them guess at and clarify these underlying assumptions and hidden meanings. For example, in exploring automatic thoughts, cognitive therapists strive to go beyond these more superficial thoughts to uncover the underlying meaning and significance to the person. That is, they strive to determine the ways of thinking that render a given experience anxiety-provoking or depressing (e.g., "Why would dying be a problem?," "If it were true that others did not like you or found you boring, how would that be significant?"). The experience and the associated emotions can *only* be understood when one is aware of the unique assumptions, preconceptions, and biases that the client brings to bear in interpreting events to determine their significance. These skills at deepening understanding are invaluable and can be integrated in the context of empathic listening to further the client's understanding of distressing events.

Others have argued that the process of good reflective listening is also therapeutic in and of itself in that it involves exposure to threatening or distressing thoughts, beliefs, and self-views (Martin, 1999). That is, clients with anxiety and depression avoid thinking about underlying threats and the negative emotions that accompany them. Emotional and experiential avoidance (e.g., suppression of imagery, affect, and emotional processing) has been identified as a key function of obsessive worrying (Borkovec & Roemer, 1995) and a key unifying characteristic underlying anxiety and mood disorders (e.g., Brown & Barlow, 2009) and all major types of mental health problems (Hayes, Strosahl, & Wilson, 2012). Martin (1999) argues that a major function of empathic listening is to heighten the client's awareness of these avoided thoughts, experiences, and emotions, thereby facilitating habituation, distress tolerance, and more adaptive ways of regulating emotion. Similarly, in discussing the role of empathy in MI for anxiety, Angus and Kagan (2009) argue that "the articulation and processing of distressing emotions within the context of a safe relational bond is a central therapeutic task when working with chronically anxious clients" (p. 1158).

Clinical Examples

Consider the following example of exploring anxious thinking with a young man with social anxiety. He initially stated that he "played to his strengths" in order to connect with women by using his attractiveness and that consequently he had few or no male friends. He was highly avoidant in his interpersonal style (e.g., making limited eye contact with me and reluctant to self-disclose), and thus I initially used empathic reflection to create safety and establish a working alliance. This excerpt comes from early in treatment (session 3) where we were beginning to understand his particular set of meanings embedded in anxiety-provoking events. The understanding of the direct role of empathy in facilitating self-confrontation and experiential awareness, outlined above, is highlighted in bracketed comments.

THERAPIST: So, if you were to decide to expand your connections with others, what would a baby step toward that look like—hypothetically? You don't have to act on it, but let's just picture it. [explicitly preserving autonomy by freeing the client from pressure to act when envisioning steps to change]

CLIENT: I'm only comfortable when I'm with women and I'm flirting. But when I'm with men or with women where I don't or can't flirt, I'm anxious. So, maybe I wouldn't flirt with a female friend.

THERAPIST: And what comes up for you as you picture that? What's the fear?

CLIENT: Oh, man, I'm anxious just thinking about it. [The client reports negative affect aroused by picturing a feared scenario; he may be only vaguely aware of his experience and the thinking underlying it; not understanding it, beyond the immediate knowledge that he feels anxious]

THERAPIST: So, it's hard even talking about it . . . picturing it. If you're willing, speak from that fear . . . what does it say? [The therapist acknowledges his currently present experience of anxiety and encourages further elaboration, that is, the exposure to feared feelings and assumptions.]

CLIENT: I won't have anything to say. There will be silence.

THERAPIST: And silence is not good . . . if you can't think of something to say, other people will see that and judge you . . . they will think you're inadequate somehow. [guessing at underlying assumptions and keeping the client in the feared experience]

CLIENT: Yeah. Like I can't even make small talk. It will be awkward and uncomfortable.

THERAPIST: So, you'll feel anxious and frightened . . . maybe they won't like you. [acknowledging experience and guessing at further meaning]

CLIENT: Or they'll think I'm boring.

THERAPIST: And then they won't want to spend time with you . . . they might reject you. [further guessing at underlying meaning]

CLIENT: Like, right now, I'm remembering a time when I was at a party, and it was just me and this other guy in the kitchen at one

point. And it was incredibly awkward. Like we didn't have anything to say to one another. We couldn't even make small talk. It
was horrible!

THERAPIST: What was going through your mind as you stood there
in that kitchen? [The therapist keeps the focus on elaboration of
experience.]

CLIENT: It was just really tense and awkward. [The client moves to
generalities and global characterizations.]

THERAPIST: And there's something bad about tense and awkward . . .
like it's not okay. [The therapist continues to encourage symboliza-
tion and elaboration of experience and guess at possible meaning
that leads him to experience the encounter as anxiety-provoking
. . . in order to deepen his understanding.]

CLIENT: Yes. I felt stupid.

THERAPIST: And if you feel stupid, then maybe you are stupid.
[Importantly, this was not offered in a spirit of challenging the
client's beliefs but rather as an elaboration of his underlying
assumptions.]

CLIENT: That's kind of harsh actually. But it certainly feels like it.

THERAPIST: Yeah. You feel incompetent, inept. And he's seeing that
and thinking that too. [further stretching awareness of experience
and elaborating the underlying assumptions]

CLIENT: Yeah. Like, I think people will broadcast that, you know.
Like, if one person sees me being awkward, then everyone will
find out.

THERAPIST: Yeah, like, that's newsworthy somehow. It's important
information for people. [Again, here the therapist is not intending
to "challenge" the client's beliefs or push for change but intending
to deepen the client's awareness of his implied assumptions so that
he can see them more clearly; note, however, that if the therapist
were intending to offer this as a suggestion for a new perspective,
he or she could freely do so but only while explicitly preserving
client autonomy; see the preceding chapter, for example, "I don't
know if this fits for you at all—but you seem to be saying that this
is important information for people").

CLIENT: (*Laughs.*) Like, I'm the center of the universe or something.
People have nothing better to worry about! [emergent nonanxious
change voice upon recognition of underlying assumptions]

THERAPIST: (*Laughs in response.*) Well, I know I get daily updates on
your interactional prowess.

CLIENT: (*Laughs in response.*) Like, I think word will spread like wild-fire!

THERAPIST: That's what your anxiety says. So, no wonder you're scared. If I thought my every foible would be broadcast news, I certainly would feel anxious too. [validation and also serves to dampen a possible self-chastising by reflecting that it's a normal response to a threatening idea] And I could be wrong about this—but I'm also hearing that maybe you don't agree or that maybe you have something else you want to say about that. [The therapist picks up on the client's laughter upon the reflection of his behavior as being newsworthy and hears this as an indication that an emergent alternative voice is beginning to object to this anxious assumption; then seeks to evoke and have *the client* elaborate this new voice or perspective; note as well that, since this is an observation of the therapist and comes from the therapist's perspective—thus, in an MI spirit—it still explicitly preserves the client's autonomy.]

CLIENT: Yes. Like, not everyone cares about what I do. Like, other people make mistakes too or have awkward moments.

THERAPIST: Like, maybe it's normal and not a huge cause for others' concern. Maybe they'll be forgiving or even understand. [reflecting and elaborating an alternative perspective, which has the impact of encouraging the client to elaborate further]

CLIENT: Yeah. Like, other people experience it too. So, they might not be so hard on me.

THERAPIST: So, there's another voice I'm hearing now that seems to be important—it's not taking the anxious voice at face value. It says, "The anxious voice is pretty extreme, and just maybe it's not always right." If it seems okay, can you speak more from that new voice? [identifying an emergent new possible perspective and seeking to have the client elaborate it further]

CLIENT: Well, I think that no one is perfect. And everyone makes mistakes. And that doesn't damn you to a lifetime of loneliness and rejection.

THERAPIST: I see. So, maybe if others are imperfect, then you can be too. Say more . . .

We spent significant time elaborating and hearing this new emergent voice while being cautious to gently encourage such expansion (undershooting reflections rather than being too enthusiastic about and pushing for the emerging alternative or change perspective). That is, the client needs to feel safe enough to expand this new, initially fragile, underdeveloped perspective and needs reassurance that the therapist will not preemptively insist on change. I also blended the integration of other interventions derived from my own perspective/external expertise with empathic listening (see Chapter 10). In particular, I offered brief psychoeducation to help the client with the task of elaborating the alternative perspective while freeing the client from pressure to act on this voice. In particular:

> "This voice sounds really new and kind of weak right now, but it sounds like it might have some important things to bring into the conversation. I could be wrong about this, but it also sounds more like you. If it feels okay to do so, it might be important to give it some airtime and hear what it is saying, because it seems to just get hijacked all the time by the anxious voice. The anxious voice might win out at the end of the day, but there may be no harm in at least hearing what the other part of you has to say. Does that sound okay?."

I also suggested that the client start writing some of these things down in the session to capture what this newly emergent perspective was saying and suggesting, and I suggested that he spend some time between sessions hearing and elaborating this new voice. Again, these suggestions were presented while reinforcing client autonomy—that is, he didn't have to "buy" or act on this new voice, but rather the exercise was just about hearing it.

Now, this may sound like basic and probably reasonably good cognitive therapy to many readers. And I, of course, agree. However, the style and underlying therapist attitude in helping the client confront existing views and ways of being is important to be explicit about. In particular, using empathic reflection in the spirit and style described by Rogers (1975) and the close attention to the moment-to-moment unfolding process both seem key. The attitude of the therapist in using empathic reflection is that understanding, elaboration, and increasing awareness are regarded as important goals in and of themselves.

Using a joined frame of reference (sometimes even reflected in the therapist's use of the pronoun *I* as opposed to *you* when speaking "as the client"), the therapist seeks to deepen the client's awareness of distressing experiences, offering or guessing at possible layers of meaning, hidden assumptions, or other facets of experience that are implicit but not yet articulated. The therapist advances these as tentative possibilities, with correction, disagreement, or revision made as needed when the client checks these guesses against his or her own experience. Even guessing wrong encourages the client to elaborate his or her experience and assumptions further. Sometimes the therapist articulates this tentativeness explicitly, for example, "Is that right?," "I'm guessing that . . . ," "If I hear you right, you're saying . . ." This communicates to the client that he or she is the sole and ultimate authority on his or her experience, with the therapist as facilitator in the service of the client's own exploration and self-understanding.

Thus, regarding this exploration as an important end in itself, the therapist takes his or her time in elaborating and seeking to understand the client's existing assumptions and experience. That is, the therapist is not exploring the client's thinking and experience because it is a necessary step for later disputation (i.e., a means to another end) but rather trusts and recognizes this exploration *as valuable in itself.* The therapist understands that when he or she is patient with this process and the client sees and more fully understands his or her own assumptions and experience, the client begins to spontaneously answer, deconstruct, and evaluate them.

In other words, self-confrontation often naturally emerges in the context of good empathic listening (persistent efforts to uncover and discover nuances and facets of the client's experience, beliefs, and assumptions and then to offer these back to the client for correction and revision). Just as staying with one side of ambivalence naturally evokes the other side, fully articulating, understanding, and validating existing sets of assumptions and coping behaviors naturally leads the client to confront them and consider alternative perspectives and approaches (i.e., "As I hear myself, there is a part of me that objects or thinks differently"). This joined frame of reference is arguably powerful in promoting client safety to explore experience further and elaborate these emergent alternative perspectives. Moreover, this process in and of itself also facilitates exposure to avoided and distressing thoughts and experiences. Taking one's time to help the client fully elaborate his or her thoughts in distressing situations is not merely a means to another end (e.g., constructing between-session experiments involving exposure) but rather constitutes exposure to feared or distressing events itself.

> *Helping the client fully elaborate his or her experience itself serves as exposure to distressing events.*

Approaching these important tasks with reflective listening in the spirit outlined by Rogers (1975) has the advantage of lowering the risk of alliance ruptures and resistance. A good example of this is when the therapist in the preceding vignette roughly states, "[your skill at conversation] is newsworthy somehow. It's important information for people." The therapist, working from an empathic listening frame, is intending this comment merely as a further guess at the client's set of assumptions and experience, which the client can then reject or affirm. The therapist has no agenda other than to know his or her clients and to help the client know themselves and see themselves more clearly. Most significantly, the therapist is *not* attempting to point out that the client's thinking is irrational or to correct him (or her) by imposing an agenda promoting change (i.e., the goal is not strategic). Any statement offered with that more strategic intent would risk evoking resistance if the client were not yet ready to consider change. When statements are offered in the MI spirit, conversely, the client can then spontaneously choose to (but doesn't have to!) confront his own experience or respond with an objection to his assumptions because his own thinking seems ridiculous *to him* as he hears it articulated more clearly and fully. In other words, it is not up to the therapist to judge (e.g., agree or disagree) or even challenge the client's experience or assumptions—that is the client's job, and the therapist can only facilitate it. As Watson et al. (1998) point out, it is only in the service of understanding that the therapist can comment on client perceptions, and it is the client who ultimately determines whether they are valid, accurate, or worthwhile.

Consider another illustration of the potential of empathic reflection to promote exposure to unwanted and avoided experience (i.e., promote experiential awareness). This client had severe health anxiety and manifested a very challenging style of intellectualizing. She spoke very quickly, moved rapidly from topic to topic, was keen on efforts to dissect and analyze her problems, and frequently asked questions of me (e.g., "Is experience *X* common?," "Where does symptom *Y* come from?," "I'm doing *Z*—is that the right thing to do?"). In general, she was highly engaged in taking steps toward recovery (e.g., reading many self-help books with some good effect, engaged with self-monitoring and other exercises that we would develop). However, many times in session I would experience her questions and topic switches as highly distracting and diverting from her experience of anxiety (e.g., as efforts to gain reassurance and certainty) and consequently diversions from the process of exposure (which she would rather talk about than do).

Over time, I shifted to the judicious use of empathy as a way of helping this client to experience unwanted and avoided feelings. For example, I worked hard to resist her efforts to problem-solve, offered observations (while supporting her autonomy) about her tendencies to switch topics, and did my best to respond to her questions with empathy rather than answers. For example:

> CLIENT: Sometimes I don't know what the right thing is to do. (*pause*) But isn't everyone like that, though? Isn't that normal?
>
> THERAPIST: You're wondering whether you're abnormal—because sometimes you feel that way. And there's a sense of "I'm not sure whether it's okay to be like that if everyone else is not like that."
>
> CLIENT: (*smiling*) That's it! I just want to fit in, you know.

THERAPIST: And you feel like you don't always fit in. And that feels like it's not okay somehow.

After persistent efforts of this kind, at various points during the sessions the client would start to cry deeply. I would then use empathy to help her stay with and explore this experience. For example:

THERAPIST: (*softly*) You're hurting. It feels very sad.

CLIENT: (*tearfully*) Yes.

THERAPIST: Speak from the tears. What are they about?

CLIENT: (*tearfully*) I don't know. (*pause*) I'm sorry.

THERAPIST: (*softly*) No need to apologize. It's okay. Take your time, and when you're ready try to say more about what you're feeling. "I feel . . . "

CLIENT: (*pause*) So sad and confused (*long pause—more tears*). What's coming up for me right now is my kids. I feel like I don't do the right thing by them sometimes—like, I am strict rather than being supportive. I just tell them what to do all the time.

THERAPIST: You have regrets. You're not sure you're the kind of parent you want to be, and that hurts.

CLIENT: (*tearfully*) Yes. It's like I feel like my job is to be in control all the time—like, that's what parents are supposed to do. Set rules. Set the right direction for their kids. But that might not be the best thing for them. I'm so worried that they might rebel and get into trouble when they become teenagers.

THERAPIST: You're trying to do the right thing—to protect them.

CLIENT: Exactly.

THERAPIST: And you're the kind of parent that others expect you to be, but maybe you're not the kind that *you* want to be. And you're really frightened about what the future could hold for your kids if you don't lighten up—be more yourself.

The client was frequently tearful throughout this discussion as she began to become more aware of her fears for her children and ambivalence about her parenting. In later sessions, she also became more open to expressing insecurities and feelings of inadequacy that she typically worked hard to hide from others (based on beliefs that others would judge her and lose respect for her). She also reflected that she was beginning to experience her continual worrying about and obsession with her health as a distraction from these other concerns (i.e., "It's like it gives me something else to think about"), which allowed her to begin to gain some distance from it. She also disclosed her fears about showing negative emotion and reported that she often resists doing so since one of her beliefs is that any display of negative affect will inevitably lead to a mental breakdown and severe depression.

Thus, the act of creating conditions through the judicious use of empathy was an exposure exercise in itself. It enabled her to gain new information about the accuracy of her belief about the implications of experiencing negative affect. As such, rather than talking about and teaching her about the necessity of not avoiding and getting in touch with unwanted feelings and fears, the heavy reliance on empathy facilitated direct access to (and ultimately working through) these painful avoided experiences. Moreover, empathic reflection accomplished this goal in a way that teaching her about these things could not achieve.

In other words, developing and integrating the core MI skill of empathic listening—even when clients are receptive to and interested in taking action to change—is a powerful tool that can be used to advance important and common treatment goals among those with anxiety and depression. Such important treatment goals include heightening self- and experiential awareness and providing important opportunities for exposure to avoided feelings, avoided self-views, and the like. In particular, the experience of a therapist embodying the core facilitative conditions outlined by Rogers (1951, 1956), including empathic understanding, is considered essential in triggering "safeness," deactivating hyperaroused threat detection systems, and creating a context that allows for exploration of distressing and painful issues (Gilbert, 1993, 2010; Gilbert & Irons, 2005). Gilbert and colleagues have further argued that generating alternative thoughts in CBT, for example, may be of limited efficacy in the absence of the experience of a soothing, caring other that the patient can internalize to promote self-soothing (Gilbert & Irons, 2005; Rector, Bagby, Segal, Joffe, & Levitt, 2000).

Unfortunately, there can be a tendency to devalue the complex and difficult skill of providing empathy (e.g., as "just listening") and consequently to underutilize it at the action stage in favor of other interventions. On the other hand, consistent with MI, empathic listening can be viewed as a potent and powerful intervention in its own right. It can achieve important objectives in helping clients overcome anxiety and related feelings of depression, and it does so with far less risk of resistance than interventions introduced from the

> *Empathic listening helps a client overcome anxiety and depression with little risk of resistance.*

therapist's frame of reference. Interpersonally, it also communicates a view of the client that is conducive to promoting client self-acceptance and self-reliance.

USING EMPATHY TO FACILITATE SELF-ACCEPTANCE

For Rogers (1951), empathic listening was central and considered a vital and powerful vehicle for communicating an underlying attitude of belief in and regard for the client and unleashing the client's potential for self-realization and change. He observed, for example:

> It would appear that for me, as a counsellor, to focus my whole attention and effort upon understanding and perceiving as the client perceives and understands, is a striking operational demonstration of the belief I have in the worth and significance of this individual client. Also the fact that I permit the outcome to rest upon this deep understanding is probably the most vital operational evidence which could be given that I have confidence in the potentiality of the individual for constructive change and development in the direction of a more full and satisfying life. (1951, p. 35)

As such, empathic listening is an important vehicle for communicating the view of the therapist toward the client—or, in the case of MI, the underlying spirit of MI. Being regarded in this way by another can be a unique and valuable experience for clients with anxiety and depression who often have long histories of being poorly regarded and maltreated by others and have internalized negative self-views and self-perceptions as a result. The therapist acceptance and nonjudgmental attitude toward the client that is reflected in empathic listening can be a powerful force in stimulating greater self-acceptance in the client. For example, Gilbert and Irons (2005) argue that "the empathic and soothing behaviors of the therapist get empathically created in the patient" (p. 296). In fact, they assert that the client's sense of self is constantly being sculpted in interaction.

Based on this perspective, clients plagued with self-criticism, shame, and self-condemnation can come to view themselves with more compassion, acceptance, and tolerance through the therapist's consistent communication and instantiation

Empathic listening stimulates client self-acceptance.

of such an alternative view. In essence, such interactions are experienced (often uncomfortably at first) as discrepant from the typical way of being treated by others and one's typical view of self. Therefore, they can be powerful antidotes to self-disregard, in and of themselves. That is, such experiences can serve as catalysts for entertaining other possible, more positive, views of self and experimenting with alternative ways of being and thinking.

For example, the client who feels unworthy of another's attention is pleasantly surprised to find that the therapist regards his or her experiences as valuable, valid, and worthy of exploration. The client with social anxiety

who harbors beliefs in the judgment of others, and who shows awkwardness at being the focus of the therapist's attention, experiences the therapist
as nonjudgmental and accepting. The client who feels terrified to demonstrate weakness in front of others cries in the presence of the therapist or
reveals other shameful experiences—and finds that, rather than being hor-
rified, the therapist values the client's courage and is eager to learn more
about his or her experience.

Thus, providing empathy can communicate powerful interpersonal
messages that violate client expectations based on existing self-views and
ways of being regarded. Such discrepancies, over time, can play an important role in causing clients to question and reexamine their existing beliefs
and self-perceptions. For clients with anxiety and related problems, these
unusual relational experiences can translate, over time, into displacing self-
hostility with greater self-regard, self-acceptance, and self-compassion.

SUMMARY

A therapeutic relationship characterized by empathy has been found to be
a powerful agent of change in therapy (Bohart, Elliott, Greenberg, & Watson, 2002; Greenberg, Elliott, Watson, & Bohart, 2001; Orlinsky, Grawe,
& Parks, 1994). For example, Burns and Nolen-Hoeksma (1992) found
that therapeutic empathy had a substantial causal effect on recovery from
depression in clients receiving CBT, even when homework compliance was
controlled. Much has been written about the value of empathy, particularly
from process–experiential and client-centered perspectives (e.g., Bohart &
Greenberg, 1997). Moreover, there is a large body of literature on correc-
tive interpersonal experiences in psychodynamic theory and contemporary
interpersonal theory (e.g., Alexander & French, 1946; Benjamin, 2003;
Kiesler, 1996).

My purpose here is not to present a comprehensive discussion of this
important topic(s). Rather, there can be a tendency to deemphasize empathic
listening in favor of more directive and action-oriented skills with clients
who are highly motivated for change. And I recommend that the MI skill
of empathic listening should not be restricted to the goal of understanding
ambivalence and building motivation but rather can be judiciously used
over the entire course of therapy. Doing so offers important advantages of
safeguarding the therapeutic alliance and reducing the probability of resistance when clients approach the important and difficult tasks of developing
new views of self, exposing themselves to unwanted and avoided experiences, and reducing self-hostility and self-judgment in favor of greater self-
acceptance.

Thus, ultimately empathic reflection can be an additional and important tool—and represent active intervention—to accomplish the critical goals common to the treatment of anxiety and depression of increasing self-awareness and helping clients deconstruct their self-views so that they can begin to critically evaluate them. Moreover, empathic listening can be a powerful vehicle for directly helping clients access and face unwanted and avoided thoughts, feelings, and experiences. To the extent that empathy communicates a different view of the client (a unique and different way of being regarded by another), it can also serve as a catalyst for greater self-acceptance and self-regard among clients with chronically low feelings of self-worth and high levels of self-criticism. Additionally, empathy has other functions as well, such as promoting self-soothing, emotional regulation, and reduced feelings of isolation (Rogers, 1975). That is, rather than considering empathic listening as mainly a supportive nondirective approach to be used in the context of resistance, this key MI skill can constitute an important and powerful intervention in its own right and should not be abandoned in favor of more directive educational methods that arise from the therapist's own frame of reference.

12

CR

Rolling with Resistance

Rolling with resistance is a key skill to integrate when encountering resistance during the action phase of therapy. It is common for clients to experience momentary objections to change or derailments in their motivation to change despite successfully having already taken some action toward change. This is a normal part of the vicissitudes of change. The familiar way of being (the status quo position) is very well rehearsed and often resurfaces, sometimes with significant force. It is important for the client to experience this in order to further consolidate his or her skills in responding effectively from the change position. At these moments, the therapist needs to shift out of facilitating action and into a more supportive position in hearing and addressing this resistance. Doing so also allows the client, rather than the therapist, to wrestle with this resistance to change.

In MI, resistance is considered to be the product of the client's ambivalence about change and how the therapist responds to this ambivalence (Moyers & Rollnick, 2002).

Respond flexibly to resistance; shift out of facilitating action, and assume a supportive position.

In order for resistance to be present, there has to be something or someone to resist, and thus the therapist plays a major role in either amplifying or diminishing resistance which is consistent with research on resistance (see Chapter 3). Sustained resistance often occurs when the therapist attempts to persuade or continues to make demands, such as advocating or pushing for change for which the client is not ready. The overriding task is to double back, genuinely seek to understand and validate the wisdom in the resistance, and reestablish harmony in the therapeutic relationship.

Thus, resistance is most often encountered when the therapist advises, directs, or makes suggestions. As mentioned previously, framing these communications in an MI style (i.e., suggesting ideas while preserving client autonomy; see Chapter 10) can be useful in increasing receptivity to therapist suggestions. However, even when framing more directive methods in the MI style, resistance can often be encountered. At these times, again the therapist needs to be prepared to back down from pushing for compliance and to shift to a more reflective and supportive stance.

SPECIFIC METHODS FOR ROLLING WITH RESISTANCE

In *Motivational Interviewing: Preparing People for Change* Miller and Rollnick (2002) describe a number of specific responses that embody the spirit of rolling with resistance. Consistent with the view elaborated more fully in Chapter 6, resistance should not viewed as something to be defeated but rather as expected and understandable, and as an important opportunity to help the client understand his or her ambivalence about change.

The specific methods for responding to (or "rolling with") resistance recommended by Miller and Rollnick (2002) are summarized in Table 12.1. These specific responses in MI are illustrated by considering possible responses to a client resistance statement in anxiety and depression, respectively.

Extended Clinical Examples

Since it is important to capture the context of the presentation of resistance in order to conceptualize how to effectively navigate resistance, below I provide four clinical illustrations of rolling with resistance. These examples capture a range of common presentations of anxiety and depression. Each of them provides illustrations of rolling with resistance with clients who are already taking action to change (i.e., are in the action phase). Commentary on what is happening moment to moment and the particular strategies the therapist uses appear in brackets.

Example 1: Generalized Anxiety Disorder

This first example illustrates the application of rolling with resistance strategies in the context of ongoing work with a client with GAD whose worry primarily centered on work. She initially had strong fears of being fired, which would lead her to become preoccupied with this possibility and spend excessive unproductive amounts of time reiterating her fears to

TABLE 12.1. Illustrations of Responses to Resistance in Anxiety
and Depression

Anxiety example: "I know I have to start conversations to get over my anxiety, but whenever I do I just end up looking stupid, and that sets me back even more."

Depression example: (on the heels of opposing a therapist suggestion) "Do you know what it's like to be depressed?"

Simple reflection. Acknowledge the person's disagreement, objection, feeling, or perception.
   Anxiety example: "You're concerned that this will makes things worse."

   Depression example: "You're wondering whether I really understand how hard this is for you to consider right now."

Amplified reflection. Reflect back what the person has said in an amplified or exaggerated form. State it in a more extreme manner.
   Anxiety example: "This can only end badly."

   Depression example: "You're wondering whether I can *ever* understand how you're feeling."

Double-sided reflection. Capture both sides of the ambivalence. If both sides are not evident in the statement, bring the absent side in through knowledge of what the client has previously said.
   Anxiety example: "Part of you knows there is probably some merit to doing this, and another part of you questions whether it's wise."

   Depression example: "I'm asking you to scale a mountain when it might make sense to start with something more sensible."

Reframing. Find something positive in what the client has said. Reframe it positively. This acknowledges the validity of the person's observations while at the same time offering a new meaning or interpretation. This is similar to Roger's concept of prizing a client—especially when he or she is opposing you or change.
   Anxiety example: "You know yourself well enough to know that it's smart to pick the right time for these types of challenges. You want to set yourself up to succeed."

   Depression example: "It's important that I understand what this is really like for you. And I couldn't agree more." Or "You know what you need and aren't afraid to say so when we get offtrack."

Agreeing with a twist. Offer acknowledgment, with a simultaneous slight twist or change of direction. This retains a sense of consonance with the client while continuing to influence the direction and momentum of change: a reflection with a reframe.
   Anxiety example: "We certainly don't want to set you up to fail. That wouldn't make any sense at all. It's important that we work together to find things that seem sensible."

TABLE 12.1. *(continued)*

Depression example: "I hear you telling me something that I need to understand and more fully appreciate—just how hard it is to do things when you feel depressed."

Emphasizing personal choice and control. Explicitly reassure the person of what the truth is; in the end it is always the client who determines what happens.
Anxiety example: "This might not be the right thing to do. Only you know what's best."

Depression example: "You're certainly the best expert on how you feel, and no one can really know what it's like to be you. I certainly fail in that effort at times and need you to remind me when I'm offtrack."

Coming alongside. When a therapist occupies the prochange position, an ambivalent client is forced to articulate the arguments for the status quo. Thus, therapists can occupy the status quo position in the context of ambivalence, which in turn ultimately encourages or helps the client to articulate the change position. Importantly, this is not a paradoxical intention which is inconsistent with MI. In coming alongside, the MI therapist is genuinely seeking to side with the client and ultimately defuse the argument.
Anxiety rexample: "It's not worth the risk to start conversations."

Depression gexample: "I can never really know what it's like to be you."

Shifting focus. Shift the person's attention away from the stumbling block. Go around barriers rather than trying to surmount them or persuade the client. This is especially useful if you feel like persuading and can't think of another response in that moment to roll with resistance (i.e., it might help move you away from taking a persuading position).
Anxiety example: "I hear that starting conversations definitely doesn't seem like the right thing to consider right now. Is there something else that might be more doable? What would be more useful for us to focus on?"

Depression example: "I make suggestions sometimes without appreciating that it's tremendously difficult, maybe impossible, to follow through with them. When we were discussing the thought record, that seemed to flow more smoothly. It might be wise to return to that. What do you think?" (In this particular instance, since the client has identified a serious therapist failing— lack of empathy—it is important to acknowledge this. Abruptly shifting focus would appear quite unempathic.)

---

others in order to get reassurance. The client was working productively toward reduced anxiety using MI-infused CBT and was highly engaged and able to access alternative, less anxiety-provoking positions as well as to reduce reassurance seeking and preoccupation with worry. In the session excerpt below, however, she reported significant anxiety that was triggered by recent events at work.

CLIENT: I saw my boss go into meetings with senior officials, and she didn't say a word to me when she came out.

THERAPIST: And that has you worried.

CLIENT: Yes, there's been a problem with a bug in a software program I wrote that customers had been complaining about. I solved it, but I'm wondering if all this has something to do with me. I've seen it before where people are just excluded from stuff and then escorted away without warning.

THERAPIST: You worry that you'll be fired. What would that mean?

CLIENT: I'd be embarrassed. It's also a tough economic climate out there right now. I might not get another job.

THERAPIST: And what would that mean?

CLIENT: I'd end up getting depressed again, which would make it even harder for me to get another job.

THERAPIST: So, your anxiety tells you that this could end really badly and spiral out of control. Sounds like a very familiar place that you've wrestled with before. I don't know if it's possible, but what might be an alternative way of thinking about this? [The therapist encourages the client to consider alternative ways of viewing the situation while preserving her autonomy.]

CLIENT: Well, the job climate *is* really tough right now. My brother, who is in the same field, has been out of work for over 2 years. And in my field, you can be 99% accurate and still get fired. Every bug leads to complaints, and the software developers get blamed for everything. [Resistance emerges. The client is opposing the therapist's agenda of countering the worry and defending the no change position. This type of exchange went on for a few minutes with no traction in developing a soothing response to the anxiety, and her resistance continued.]

THERAPIST: It's almost like it makes sense to be proactive here . . . to entertain the possibility that you might be fired, because it helps you prepare for what might happen. It sounds like it would be naive to live in the fantasy where this isn't a real possibility. [The therapist is rolling with resistance; reframing and coming alongside; guessing at advantages or good reasons for the client's remaining anxious.]

CLIENT: Yes, absolutely. It protects me.

THERAPIST: It's like a useful coping strategy to think ahead and envision the disasters that might happen. (*pause*) Maybe you should think about polishing up your resume. [The therapist continues to roll with resistance by using reframing and is also validating the client's underlying need to feel protected by anticipating future possible negative events.]

CLIENT: Yes, I know it's possible to get fired. [The client then reiterates the reasons for catastrophic thinking and resisting change. But note that interpersonally the therapist and the client are no longer struggling or at cross-purposes. The client is cooperating with the therapist's revised agenda of understanding resistance to change.]

THERAPIST: So, it's even kind of weird to call these thoughts "anxiety"— this is a necessary survival strategy in a cutthroat industry. [The therapist is continuing to roll with resistance, reframing anxiety as not a bad thing but a good thing, i.e., the therapist is empathically following by reflecting what is alive for the client in that moment—the value of anxious thinking.]

CLIENT: Well (pause), I'd still call it "anxiety" actually. I tend to take it too far . . . to the point where I start to drive myself and others nuts. I need to be less anxious about things like this. [Change talk begins to reemerge; having "heard" her position of the value in worry as empathically reflected by the therapist, the client begins to reevaluate its utility and appraise the need for other strategies to cope with this situation.]

THERAPIST: So, it protects you to anticipate the negative things that could happen. And you're good at that . . . you need to do that to some extent. But you also need to put the brakes on that kind of thinking at times . . . take it down a notch. [Double-sided reflection captures the totality of the client's current position. Also, the therapist takes care to not "jump" too hastily to the emerging change position by reiterating a key function of the no-change position and softly supporting the change position through such phrases as "at times" and "take it down a notch." This makes it easier for the client to respond with more change talk. If the therapist had used reflections that were too far ahead of the client's current position such as "I have to stop this anxiety!," this would likely have elicited resistance and defense of the no-change position.]

CLIENT: Yes. I need to hold it in check. [The client reiterates the need for change.]

THERAPIST: Why? [The therapist is seeking to elaborate and consolidate reemerging arguments for change.]

CLIENT: Because I blow things out of proportion and make myself and other people miserable.

THERAPIST: And you want and need to be able to respond in a more balanced way . . . a way that is less catastrophic and dire. So, in this situation, if you were to consider "holding it in check," what might that look like? [The therapist uses tentative language to reinforce client autonomy but follows the emerging change talk and seeks to elaborate it.]

CLIENT: Well, for one thing, I will get another job. I know that. And my boss's behavior could be about something that has nothing to do with me. There's nine of us in the same position as me; so, even if it is about software, the odds are only one in nine that it's about me.

THERAPIST: And those are pretty good odds.

CLIENT: Yes. And I do do good work. I did fix this problem. So, even if they downsize me, it's not a reflection on my skill.

THERAPIST: There's no need to be embarrassed here.

CLIENT: It would be their loss.

Here, the therapist initially continues with the change agenda since this client had been successfully taking action to develop more adaptive alternative responses to worry. However, on hearing the client's repeated resistance to change, the therapist stops pursuing change and shifts to getting alongside of and more fully elaborating and understanding the counterchange position. In interpersonal process terms, the client's resistance is communicating, "I'm not listening to you. At this moment, I'm not on the same page as you. I'm not willing to follow where you are leading right now." That is, resistance is simply a type of stop signal (Miller & Rollnick, 2002). It reflects vitally important information about engagement, namely, that the therapist is not appreciating something important that the client is attempting to communicate or bring into the conversation. The therapist needs to hear this message and go where the client is. Hearing the arguments for not changing reflected and validated by the therapist frees the client to determine for herself which response to the current stressor makes the most sense for her.

Note that this type of flexibility is very difficult to master in my experience, since the therapist can become attached to or immersed in facilitating change and have difficulty shift-

> Resistance indicates that the therapist is not hearing something important that the client is trying to communicate.

ing to *genuinely* hearing the reemergent arguments for not changing. This flexibility is especially difficult to master if one is used to and well practiced at advocating for change or predominantly used to being on the side of the prochange position. For example, in this case, the therapist experienced a sense of "disappointment" at hearing the client resist change, especially since the client had been working so well to accomplish change. Initially, the therapist had pressured the client to change as a way of responding to and relieving their own feelings and sense of disappointment. Thus, the therapist had to do the internal work of subordinating her own feelings, reactions, and wishes in order to reengage and join with the client.

Example 2: Obsessive–Compulsive Disorder

In many cases where clients have already taken some action toward change, they require only a temporary shift by the therapist in considering the merits of the counterchange position before reengaging with change, that is, deciding that they prefer change. Consider the following example of the client mentioned earlier who devoted copious amounts of time to pondering thoughts about the future in an effort to gain certainty about possible courses of action but who had been successfully limiting these thoughts. In this session, she articulated arguments for not continuing to reduce obsessing about the future.

CLIENT: Yeah, but part of me feels like I'm wasting time when I don't think about what could happen. I'm not being productive.

THERAPIST: It could very well be a waste of time. What do you think? [rolling with resistance using amplified reflection and reinforcing client autonomy and freedom of choice]

CLIENT: Well, it's spending time on myself. So, in that sense it's productive in a different way. [change talk]

THERAPIST: And how important is that? You might feel that it's not appropriate to spend time on yourself. [The therapist specifically softens the invitation to elaborate change talk in order to increase the probability of client receptivity to elaborating this position and reduce the probability of further resistance.]

CLIENT: Actually, it's very important. I think that not spending time on myself is a big part of the reason I'm unhappy.

THERAPIST: So, if I'm hearing you right, even though you have to work to get around the OCD's objections, it might be worth persisting with. Is that right?

Note that the therapist's rolling with resistance ironically moves the client toward greater rearticulation of the change position. In contrast, if the therapist had advocated for the merits of the change perspective (which even the client herself previously recognized), this would place the client in the position of continuing to elaborate the merits of the nonchange position. However, rolling with resistance is *not* strategic or a type of paradoxical intervention. It is not some clever manipulation or trickery of the client so that he or she will go along with the therapist's "real" agenda of pursuing change. To engage in this type of strategic thinking would be inconsistent with the spirit of MI and reflect the attitude that the therapist knows what is best for the client. It would undermine the MI spirit of preservation of client autonomy and client self-determination. And, as I elaborated in Chapter 2, rolling with resistance (or any other MI method) is ineffective if the client-centered spirit underlying MI is not captured and genuinely inhabited by the therapist.

Example 3: Major Depression

Consider the example of a woman dealing with major depression and excessive worry. She was actively engaged in MI-infused CBT, creating an exposure hierarchy, and actively doing exposure and behavioral activation exercises between sessions with significant benefit, and in general she was highly receptive to guidance and direction. Suddenly at one session she presented as very exasperated with herself and her continued anxiety and depression. The therapist identified and reflected a strong tendency in the client toward self-criticism and a general lack of tolerance and patience, and she suggested the client consider taking a more compassionate approach to herself.

CLIENT: But why do I continue to get anxious? I hate this! It's so depressing. I try and try, but I still end up getting panicked.

THERAPIST: "It feels like I'm working so hard, I'm doing everything! But I'm not really getting anywhere." [empathic reflection communicating that the therapist hears the client's frustration]

CLIENT: I just keep having these anxious reactions again and again. It just doesn't stop!

THERAPIST: I'm also hearing you be very hard on yourself. When you speak like this to or about yourself, you get very animated, very harsh. It's like you're whipping yourself . . . beating yourself up. In my experience, that can make it a lot harder to get to where you want to be. I wonder if it might be worth considering lightening up a bit . . . being more supportive, kinder to yourself . . . cutting yourself some slack. It might be worth thinking about— but only you can know. [The therapist makes a suggestion for change.]

CLIENT: But, I should be better by now! [resistance to the suggestion and persistence with the self-critical style]

THERAPIST: And to cut yourself some slack is not appropriate here—that wouldn't help. [rolling with resistance]

CLIENT: (*speaking very adamantly*) I can do that for others, but when it comes to me it's not going to happen. It's not right!

THERAPIST: Just out of curiosity, why would you do that for others? [Note here that the therapist is continuing to advocate for change and not hearing the client's central message that she is unwilling to be more compassionate toward herself; the therapist is torn between pushing for change and rolling with resistance.]

CLIENT: Because it's not nice to criticize. It's hurtful.

THERAPIST: And maybe it hurts you too when you do it to yourself? [The client cooperates with answering the therapist's question, and the therapist continues to push for a more compassionate self-view but is selectively hearing i.e., not hearing the client's objections to this.]

CLIENT: Yes, but when it comes to me, I can't let up. [Continued resistance; pushing action is not working.]

THERAPIST: It might be okay for others, but it's not a good option for you. It's just not right. And I'm guessing that it's probably helped in getting you to where you want to be. How much would you say it's helped on a scale of 0% to 100%? [rolling with resistance, reframing and exploring it—examining it for its merits]

CLIENT: 90% or better. [Here, the client probably overestimates her belief in this simply because the therapist has not yet adequately demonstrated that she has backed off from advocating for change.]

THERAPIST: So, this is an important strategy in helping you to achieve relief from all these terrible feelings. It makes sense that you would be reluctant to give that up. And it almost feels like there might be something dangerous about letting up. Would that be right? [i.e., "What's good about not changing?"]

CLIENT: Yes. Then I might as well give up.

THERAPIST: You wouldn't want to work hard anymore. You'd become lazy. So, this is motivating . . . it's keeping you going in the important fight against anxiety/depression. [rolling with resistance; reframing, i.e., finding the positive motive underlying it]

CLIENT: (*pause*) My parents . . . my mom especially always says, "Stop sniveling . . . stop whining . . . you're just feeling sorry for your-self. When you focus and don't give in to it, that's when you'll get better."

THERAPIST: [speaking as the client's mother] "I don't want to hear it. Just stop it! If you only pushed yourself harder, you wouldn't have this problem."

CLIENT: I actually don't even bother telling my parents anymore.

THERAPIST: So, you can't share your suffering . . . how much it hurts . . . how hard it is . . . it's not safe. [empathic reflection]

CLIENT: I feel judged, kind of blamed, punished. The only times I talk about it is in here and with my brother.

THERAPIST: So, on the one hand, "not letting up" really helps because it's motivating or gives you determination, but I also hear you say-ing that "sometimes when I get treated that way I can also find it deflating . . . hurtful. Rather than feeling propped up, I feel beaten down." [developing discrepancy]

CLIENT: (Nods head, pauses.) But it's not my fault.

THERAPIST: You didn't decide to be in pain like this. Maybe you do deserve some sympathy . . . some support. [empathic reflection—guessing at what is being communicated]

CLIENT: Some understanding . . . you know . . . (tearful)

THERAPIST: What does that mean?

CLIENT: Understanding of what I'm going through . . . how hard it is . . . how hard I'm trying . . . not criticism . . . not punishment. Like sometimes . . . I don't know . . . I may need something else too beyond pressure. (pause) But I can't even fathom that though—lightening up—it just feels wrong.

THERAPIST: So, you might need some compassion, some understand-ing . . . but at the same time it's hard to let that in . . . to make that change. (pause) That makes a lot of sense to me that you would have trouble with that because all you've known is the criti-cal, pushy style. You learned that well. [double-sided reflection capturing totality of the client's ambivalence; also validating the sense of wrongness and unfamiliarity of change]

CLIENT: Right. I've had that in spades.

THERAPIST: And you're probably not sure if it would help. Why would you be sure? That only stands to reason, because you have no experience with it. In fact, it might not help. [rolling with resis-tance: coming alongside]

CLIENT: I worry that it won't, but I think it might be worth a try. [change talk]

THERAPIST: So, you're not quite sure. To push or to let up—hard to decide. You don't have any evidence that letting up would help, but there's a part of you that suspects it might . . . that you might need or want some more support. But the "not letting up" style is what you've been doing, and it might be responsible for getting you to where you are now, and it might be dangerous to give that up. If you are willing, let's see if we can do some projecting on what will happen if you do or don't let up. (*The client nods.*) Where would you say you are now on a scale of 1 to 10, with 1 being "at my worst" and 10 being "where I want to be"?

CLIENT: Four or 5.

THERAPIST: So, it is helping . . . the not letting up. Slow and steady wins the race! [rolling with resistance to change]

CLIENT: Actually, no. I got to where I am because of the work I'm doing. [Change talk emerges.]

THERAPIST: Say more. [seeking to elaborate emergent change talk]

CLIENT: Well, I'm working away on those lists we made [i.e., exposure hierarchy and behavioral activation list], practicing the deep breathing, setting aside time to worry . . . that sort of thing.

THERAPIST: So, you're improving because of the actions you're taking to cope with your feelings . . . because of your courage. You're improving in spite of "not letting up," not because of it. (*The client nods; pause.*] And where would you imagine you would be in a month or two if you continued with the "not letting up" style? [empathic reflection; question offered not to convince the client of the merits of change but in the spirit of further client exploration of the possibility of change]

CLIENT: Exactly where I am now.

THERAPIST: Ouch! So, your sense is that if you keep this up you won't be any closer to where you so desperately want to be. You're not sure that letting up would help, but you're willing to try it. Is that right—does that capture what you're saying . . . where you're at?

Following this exchange, the therapist evocatively helped the client identify what "letting up" would look like for her. The client indicated that she had no idea. In this instance, the client needed help in identifying "how" to change. Drawing on the outstanding work of Paul Gilbert on self-compassion (e.g., Gilbert, 2005, 2009), the therapist suggested that she spend some time developing a perfect nurturer image and utilize her skill at "knowing what to say to others" to help develop the characteristics and responses of this hypothetical person. Further, recognizing that accepting the soothing and wisdom of such an image would be difficult for this client and that she might experience resistance to this, the therapist suggested that the client simply work on developing the image while freeing herself from the pressure to accept or act on the attendant recommendations or guidance. The client was very receptive to these suggestions and reported in the next session that she was practicing and benefiting from using self-compassion, accepting her struggle, and self-soothing in response to her emotional pain.

Again, it was difficult for me to back off from advocating for integration of self-compassion with this client since I strongly believe in and am very attached to the merits of compassion through my own personal and professional experience. Interestingly, it was only when I was able to bracket these biases and open up to, understand, and accept the merits of the client's noncompassionate approach from her perspective (and consistently communicate this understanding/acceptance) that the client felt free to begin to examine an alternative view or approach for herself.

Clients cannot simply adopt the therapist's view or preferred approach to problem resolution no matter how beneficial doing so might seem to the therapist. Rather, clients have to decide for themselves. And therapists can best facilitate this process not by pushing harder for their own perspective or preferences but rather through their willingness to genuinely hear the client's resistance, empathically follow, respect client autonomy (even when the client's thinking and decisions go against what the therapist wants or believes), and help clients consider and weigh the merits of each position for themselves and from their own perspective, values, and objectives. This challenges therapists at times to genuinely hear and embody positions and attitudes that may diverge—sometimes sharply—from their own. In these cases, it is crucial to remember that the goal is empathic understanding of the client's perspective, not agreement or disagreement with that perspective.

> *Clients have to decide for themselves—they cannot simply adopt the therapist's viewpoint.*

Example 4: Suggesting a Highly Challenging Exposure Exercise for Health Anxiety

Another common point at which resistance is encountered, in even a highly cooperative client, is when suggesting more advanced exercises such as interoceptive exposure in panic (i.e., deliberately producing feared body sensations) or worry exposure in GAD (deliberately detailing, contemplating, and sitting with the anxiety associated with thinking about one's worst-case scenario). Clients often experience these suggested exercises as counterintuitive, often initially objecting to them, and they normally need time and space to warm up to them. Consider the following example of a client with health anxiety for whom the therapist suggested worry exposure and verbal statements inviting her worst-case scenario.

THERAPIST: There's an exercise that we recommend when people are at the stage that you are at [i.e., having achieved some good worry control]. Would you like to hear more about it?

CLIENT: Sure.

THERAPIST: What we suggest people do is, instead of trying not to think of something, actively invite it in, in order to see what happens. So, for example, you could deliberately think about getting sick . . . the worst-case scenario . . . step by step. [The therapist further elaborates the worry exposure rationale.] Or, if you feel really gutsy, you might even court the worst-case scenario by saying out loud "I hope I have cancer" or "I hope I die soon."

CLIENT: (*Shudders.*) I could never do that. That would be like inviting disaster. Somehow I feel like if I really think about what could happen, then I'm actually making it more likely that it will happen. [resistance]

THERAPIST: So, it's possible that you can keep bad things from happening if you just don't think about them. [rolling with resistance; again, spirit is critical here; the therapist has to genuinely make this statement and does so simply to reflect what the client has said, i.e., to show empathy; the therapist's own belief regarding the truth or falsity of this statement is regarded as irrelevant to the goal of understanding the client's perspective]

CLIENT: But I know that's ridiculous because if that were true I would have won the lottery by now (*Laughs.*) [change talk]

THERAPIST: So, it feels untrue on some level that your thoughts control events. How much do you believe that on a scale of 1 to 100? [attempting to nurture change talk]

CLIENT: Only about 25%.

THERAPIST: Why only 25%? [encouraging further change talk]

CLIENT: Because I know it's just superstitious nonsense (*pause*), but somehow it feels wrong to flirt with disaster. [resistance]

THERAPIST: Even though you know it's probably not true that your thoughts control events, maybe it gives you a sense of control. Like the reality is that when we really look at it, we have virtually no control over the horrific events in our lives—cancer, tornados, accidents. But the anxiety says that there is something you can do—just don't think about it. That makes sense. [rolling with resistance; guessing at a possible good reason underlying resistance in order to reframe it]

CLIENT: Yes, that's it. It's empowering somehow. But I really don't have control, do I? (*pause*) Let's try this worst-case scenario thing.

Again, when the therapist demonstrates a willingness to hear the understandable and expected part of the client's objections to the suggestion and shows a willingness to explore these while explicitly preserving the client's autonomy to decide, the client is more likely to err on the side of seriously considering the suggestion. Again, this is not because the therapist is tricking the client into cooperating, but rather the client is more likely to seriously consider therapist input, advice, and suggestions when free from pressure to change because there is a part of him or her that inherently wants to change; and this part is more likely to emerge when the client fully realizes that he or she does not *have* to agree or change in order to please the therapist.

HOMEWORK NONCOMPLIANCE

Helping clients conceptualize and implement change plans between sessions is a common practice in many therapy approaches. Completion of such homework assignments is considered a major mechanism of change and thus critical to the beneficial effects of some treatments, such as CBT. For example, I recall a prominent CBT colleague using a medical metaphor to illustrate his approach to underscoring the importance of homework completion "Just as a doctor can't treat an infection if you don't take your antibiotics, I can't help you with your anxiety unless you do the homework." Having a way of managing impasses created by homework noncompliance is important in this context, particularly since homework nonadherence is very common (e.g., Helbig & Fehm, 2004). Much has been written about the methods for improving compliance and adherence in an effort to boost the efficacy of action-oriented therapies.

Using MI to inform the integration of homework activities involves cultivating particular sensitivity to the context (when and how) in which such activities are contemplated and constructed as well as assessing client engagement with such tasks. The suggestions offered in this book for cultivating MI spirit (in Chapter 2), building resolve for change (Part III), being evocative and preserving client autonomy in constructing proposed change steps (Chapters 9 and 10), continually monitoring client resistance (Part II), and responding flexibly in the context of client's lack of engagement with a task or exercise (i.e., rolling with resistance) can all be used to increase the probability of a client's successfully engaging with such tasks. They also offer guidance on how to sustain therapeutic momentum if the client is not ready to engage with the specific action steps that are proposed.

Terms such as *homework assignment* and *compliance* are consistent with and emerge from a therapist-as-expert framework. Thus, working to cultivate and integrate the spirit of MI into treatment can provide an important alternative way of thinking about such issues and, importantly, can also help avoid the impasses and loss of momentum that are often created by client "noncompliance." For example, taking steps to change or statements reflecting receptivity to and active interest in such steps often emerge from effective work in building the client's resolve to change. That is, the steps to accomplish and instantiate change (i.e., the right thing[s] to do) often become clear when clients have resolved ambivalence about changing and are clearer on their most valued directions for change. Then, building on what the client's have already started and helping them to envision and implement continuing steps in the direction of change proceed much more smoothly.

Client homework noncompliance often represents a major threat to the therapeutic alliance, in my experience, when conceptualized from a therapist-as-expert framework. There can be an overreliance on action in such approaches, with other skills being less prominent such as building client resolve, preserving client autonomy, empathic reflection, and the like. This emphasis on action often sets the stage for client resistance and noncompliance. That is, *insisting* on change, however well intentioned, makes it less rather than more likely that the client will seriously engage with the recommended homework task. For example, prior to learning MI, I recall working with a client in a CBT group for managing depression who repeatedly refused to identify and complete homework activities. We would often wrestle with each other in a futile effort to get her to do the homework. In a later treatment session, I was finally "successful" in getting her to complete a homework task. However, on that occasion she proudly announced that "I completed the homework, and it made me worse!"

Thus, a focus on establishing and achieving compliance often creates a dangerous tug of war between the client and the therapist that often ends in stalemate or, more typically, with the client emerging as the victor. And, as we have seen, pushing for change in the context of client resistance is an effective way of creating more resistance, often alienating clients in the process and stalling their progress. In such situations, even if the thera-

pist is "successful" in persuading the
client to engage with the homework
activity, such reluctant compliance
or acquiescence is won at the cost of
potentially undermining the client's
autonomy and self-determination.

*A focus on achieving
compliance can create a
dangerous tug of war.*

This outcome risks jeopardizing the therapeutic alliance, on which so much
depends. Moreover, taking action in the face of a client's lack of belief in
the value of such steps is likely a futile exercise.

In contrast, failure to engage in or follow through with action steps to
change, from an MI perspective, can be seen as providing valuable information about client readiness, which the MI therapist is continuously monitoring. There is also evidence that early signals of in-session resistance strongly
predict later homework noncompliance in CBT (Aviram & Westra, 2010).
Therefore, systematically monitoring and assessing client readiness from
the beginning of therapy can prevent or avoid problems with noncompliance that emerge later.

Rolling with and reframing such reluctance and resistance to taking
action represent important opportunities to learn more about the client's
concerns about change and when best to shift (temporarily or more exten-
sively) to working with them on understanding these concerns and building motivation. For example, noncompliance could signal high levels of
ambivalence about change—and thus indicate the need to use skills for
building motivation. Alternatively, it could signal that the client doesn't buy
the model or framework that the therapist is suggesting—therefore indicating the need for an open discussion of ways of working together and adapting these to better suit client needs. Or, noncompliance could mean that
there is a problem in the therapy relationship—and indicate a need to shift
to empathic listening to understand and work to resolve these concerns. In
any case, seeking to understand events such as homework noncompliance
as important information to help inform the therapy (rather than as problems to be defeated) is likely to be a more productive approach to sustaining
client engagement with and investment in treatment.

Clinical Example

Let me share an anecdote that enhanced my own belief in the potential
promise of responding to homework noncompliance with MI spirit and
methods. In one of my former positions I was part of an anxiety and mood
disorders treatment team in a local hospital that provided group-based
CBT. My colleagues on this team were continually struggling with and
complaining about issues of client homework noncompliance, specifically

the unacceptably large number of treatment nonresponders, owing to their lack of engagement. At that time, I was just beginning to learn MI and adapt it to the treatment of anxiety and depression. Along with me, the other therapists on the team were learning about and playing with integrating MI. We would discuss this frequently and explore the possible application of these methods in case rounds. I told them that I wanted to more intensively pilot what we were learning with some specific cases, namely, with their most noncompliant clients and the treatment nonresponders in their groups. I asked them to send such clients my way so that I could further experiment with and evaluate whether MI helped for our clients with anxiety and depression. They were thrilled about the prospect of having another option for these clients and being able to remove them from their groups (since their noncompliance often slowed down the pace and momentum of the group, and other group members would join in with the therapist's efforts to persuade clients to complete homework).

Six months after my request, such cases were only trickling in, however. Puzzled, I asked my colleagues what happened to all the folks they were struggling with in the groups and eager to refer to me. They told me that it wasn't that they were not referring such clients to me but rather that there just didn't seem to be as many such clients to refer. When I asked them to describe how they responded to homework noncompliance, they said that it was something like this:

"That is no problem at all, Mary, that you didn't do the homework. That is really common and likely just means that our timing is off. It may not make sense to do X right now. In fact, feeling torn about doing homework—even though I know there is a part of you that wants to do it—is very normal and common. This kind of treatment is really action-oriented—homework is a big part of it. So, it may not be the right match for you right now. You can choose to stay with the group—if you think that there might be some value in it for you and if there are other steps you might take or other kinds of homework that make more sense for you right now. However, this might not be the case, and only you can know. And if you decide that this type of group is not a good fit for you right now, we have another option for a treatment that helps people get ready for groups like this. What would you like to do?"

Not surprisingly, perhaps, most noncompliant clients elected to stay in the group and ended up engaging productively with it (with clinicians simply reiterating this type of response if noncompliance persisted). In essence, these therapists were integrating MI into the action phase of therapy (or at least within an action-oriented treatment program). I strongly suspect that knowing and believing in an alternative way of navigating such situations helped get *the therapists* unstuck. That is, they knew there was a viable alternative to the very stressful prospect of wrestling with clients about homework. I further suspect that the therapists had different methods and skills and a different (more compas-

> *Successful therapists know there is a viable alternative to wrestling with clients about homework.*

sionate, tolerant, empathic) framework for thinking about and navigating noncompliance once they invoked the benefits of MI in their approach.

While such anecdotal evidence does not constitute valid scientific support (and future research needs to more systematically investigate the merit of the recommendations for integrating MI into work in the action phase), it does potentially reflect the promise of such an integration in more productively engaging clients in therapy in the face of common impasses such as homework noncompliance.

SUMMARY

A major strength of MI, in my opinion, is the view that it offers therapists for thinking about resistance and, consequently, the methods that emerge from this view (the MI spirit) for productively working with it (rather than against it). Most critically, integrating MI provides a nonpejorative way of viewing resistance. In MI, issues like noncompliance and resistance are not considered to be a fault or a failing of clients. Rather, the therapist plays a vitally important role in either amplifying or diminishing client resistance. That is, resistance is not considered a client problem but a clinician skill error. Moreover, resistance also does not reflect that the therapist is misguided, wrong, inept, or has no potential to be helpful; rather, it merely indicates that one's timing is off. That is, while it is important to not be pejorative toward clients in the face of resistance, it is also important to not be pejorative toward ourselves as therapists. Rather, resistance is merely information—a signal. It reflects vital feedback that indicates a need for the therapist to be flexible in his or her methods and reactions.

While taking responsibility for this is challenging, it can also be very empowering since it offers the therapist some degree of control over managing the impasses that can often threaten to derail good therapeutic work. Integrating MI skills throughout treatment can prevent the power struggles and therapeutic impasses that can be created by noncompliance and resistance, and it offers therapists productive strategies for more effectively navigating resistance to build or sustain client momentum for change. Again, a key element in using these methods effectively is to cultivate and nurture the spirit underlying MI so that you can genuinely convey and express this more positive, supportive, and understanding view of resistance.

PART V

Putting It All Together

13

∝

Integrated Case Example

CASE DESCRIPTION

Frank is a 31-year-old man who presented with chronic, excessive, uncontrolled worry with accompanying chronic low mood (dysthymia). He reported the onset of excessive worry at age 15, with increasing salience of worry symptoms during the past 4 years. He reported worrying constantly about work, his finances, his parents' well-being, and even minor matters. A particular concern for him was his performance at work in sales and marketing for a pharmaceutical company. He reported worrying about losing accounts, pleasing customers, overall performance, and his boss's impression of his abilities and job performance. Frank reported daily experiencing many physical symptoms of anxiety, including restlessness, being easily fatigued, irritability, muscle tension, loss of concentration, and difficulty sleeping. Frank's scores on measures of worry were in the severe range and above the 90th percentile, compared to the general population. His symptoms were consistent with diagnoses of GAD and dysthymia.

Frank also reported suffering with chronically low mood for the past 3 years, including very low energy, amotivation, and increased appetite, with frequent feelings of pessimism about the future (e.g., "Why bother with things, because they won't turn out good"), and he was tearful at times during the initial interview. He noted that his anxiety and depressed mood often made him miss work for several days at a time since he would frequently feel overwhelmed and needed to "shut down." His scores on measures of depression and stress were also in the severe range.

Frank had never been married and had no children. He was cohabiting with his partner of 3 years. He described this relationship as generally supportive, although he often felt like a burden to her because of his emotional problems. He reported experiencing "lots of violence and fear growing up." In particular, he reported that his father was physically abusive to him and his mother. His parents separated when he was 12 years of age. He also reported a past history of a major depressive episode following his parents' separation. He sought psychotherapy on one previous occasion for 30 sessions but reported experiencing few benefits from the therapy.

ASSESSING READINESS FOR CHANGE

In the initial interview, Frank expressed a substantive desire to overcome his anxiety. In particular, he stated that he no longer enjoyed anything, since "worrying is my full-time job"; he rated himself as being highly distressed about his worry—at 9.8 out of 10, with 10 being "extremely distressed." He was particularly distressed about the lack of any joy in his life and how he is "never happy." However, despite this strong desire to feel better, when asked about his ideas about what steps would bring about anxiety relief, he had no reply apart from "I have no idea, because nothing has worked so far." He made frequent "I can't" statements with respect to change (e.g., "I can't imagine what would help," "I can't seem to stop worrying at all"). When asked about what steps he had taken to change, Frank exhibited resistance to my suggestion that he might build on a strategy that he had identified as potentially useful; being quick to dismiss this. For example:

> CLIENT: When things do turn up in a positive way, I can say to myself, "You worried too much about that. And the outcome is so good, and look at all that energy you spent on worrying. Next time remind yourself not to worry." [change talk]
>
> THERAPIST: So, it might be important to remind yourself of those times . . . maybe a log you could keep or something when things turn out unexpectedly well.
>
> CLIENT: (*dismissively*) Sure, yeah . . . if I could. But then I would worry about the log. [resistance to change; challenge/disagree, hopeless/complain; counterchange talk]

When asked about his outcome expectations (i.e., "How much do you expect to improve in treatment on a scale of 1 to 100%?"), he rated his expectancy for improvement at 50%. When asked why 50% and not 10%, he reported, "I think treatment is worth a try. Why not? I have nothing to lose. It seems to help other people." He also quickly noted however (and without prompting) that his worry was so entrenched that treatment would not likely benefit him [counterchange talk]. He also noted that he had been in treatment in the past with no appreciable benefit [counterchange talk]. When his experience in this past treatment was further explored, it appeared to be cognitive-behavioral or action-oriented in nature, and Frank described that the therapist had become frustrated with him because he "had trouble doing the exercises." In short, Frank appeared highly ambivalent about treatment and change, with strong desire, on the one hand, and strong skepticism about being able to change, on the other. Given this, I decided to begin with MI and provided a rationale for this that Frank seemed responsive to, acknowledging that "I find it really hard to change. I want to, but I just keep worrying anyway."

UNDERSTANDING AMBIVALENCE AND BUILDING RESOLVE

I helped Frank explore the pros and cons of worry, his particular worry related to behaviors (e.g., excessive planning, overpreparation, reassurance seeking). The following is an extended excerpt that begins in the middle of the first MI session. It illustrates the application of a number of the MI methods previously described and, most importantly, the spirit of MI. Beyond empathic listening, which is the dominant method used in this example, other specific MI strategies are highlighted in brackets. These also include what I was thinking at different points in order to illustrate how the therapist works to cultivate and maintain MI spirit and to reframe resistance to change in his or her own mind.

THERAPIST: So, if we were to look at the upsides and the downsides of worry. If we can look at it that way. What are some of the upsides of worry? You mentioned a sense of control . . . [attempting to understand resistance to change; prompting the client with a previous statement to encourage such exploration]

CLIENT: A sense of control . . . It's so hard to see anything beyond that because that's just so powerful.

THERAPIST: It's so important.

CLIENT: Yeah, because I'm on it. Don't worry. I'm already thinking what you're going to be thinking.

THERAPIST: That feeling of control is so important. Can you say more about that? [encouraging further understanding through empathic reflection followed by a specific invitation to elaborate]

CLIENT: If you can control things you can do better . . . be better. You can be the best you can be.

THERAPIST: Maximize your potential . . .

CLIENT: (*speaking quickly and forcefully*) I feel like I'm the only one in control of my life. There is no fate. There is no destiny. I take the reins. And everything I do impacts everything that will be done. And it better be done right! And I know that's out to lunch. I'm just beating myself up. That's just silly. But that's why control is so important to me. Because I think bad things, good things can happen, but at the end of the day it's my decision . . . It's my actions that impact my life.

THERAPIST: (*with emphasis*) And this is important. And there's a lot on the line here. And you're the one who has to live with this at the end of the day. [Capturing the essence of the client's adamantly delivered message; notice that even though there is a slight bit of change talk here—"I know it's out to lunch"-it is clearly not the main intent of the message.]

CLIENT: It's my choice . . .

THERAPIST: So, if you have to worry a little bit, well then, that's just the way it is. [validation—communicating that it makes perfect sense to worry, given the beliefs/context described]

CLIENT: The price I pay. Exactly!

THERAPIST: Absolutely. There's so many positive things in that. And isn't that wonderful, to want to be in control [prizing, affirming]

CLIENT: Yeah?

THERAPIST: That's a basic human need. Controllability and predictability are two huge human needs. We want to know what's going to happen, and we want to be in control of it. Even if it's bad. If we can get a sense of at least I know when that bad thing is going to happen . . . [validation—link to common humanity]

CLIENT: Then I can be prepared and control it a bit more.

THERAPIST: Absolutely. It gives you a sense of . . . my success depends on this. You need to have control, because if you're not in control . . . [validation—you are just doing something that helps you meet important needs]

CLIENT: It could get worse. Or I'll just be screwed.

THERAPIST: What would come up for you if you gave up control? If you said "I'm just going to let life do whatever life does . . . " [continuing the exploration of resistance to change by asking "What's bad about change?"]

CLIENT: Well, then I might as well give up.

THERAPIST: It feels like a resignation . . . like a defeat [reflection—also contains the implicit message "No wonder, who wants to feel defeated?"]

CLIENT: (*speaking forcefully*) What am I here for, then? Saying "Whatever happens happens, and I'll just deal with it" feels so weak to me! Like, step up to the plate. Do what you need to do . . . do what you're capable of . . . fix it or be proactive or do damage control.

THERAPIST: (*with emphasis*) Yes. And thinking ahead is a part of that. Like, thinking about what could happen is part of the way you ensure success. [Validation by linking—a lot of the behaviors you have mentioned make sense to do in view of these important underlying issues of being successful—it all fits together—it's a coherent effort to meet vital, understandable needs.]

CLIENT: Absolutely. They're tied together.

THERAPIST: If you can think about it and plan it out, then you can make sure you're not weak. [validation—"You're just trying to feel powerful"] It's a strong thing! [prizing, affirming]

CLIENT: I'm ready and able. And then I'll be prepared for what might happen.

THERAPIST: Yeah. Because what might happen if you're not prepared? I know you can't think of everything that might happen. But what might happen if you don't think of things ahead of time . . . don't worry? [exploring resistance further by asking "What's bad about change?"]

THERAPIST: Well, then, I'm the annoying person who forgot to bring the form to the meeting that's critical. But if I worry about it enough, I'll put it in its to-go box. Or, on another level, so I'm late paying my bill, no big deal, it will get paid. But then, when I want to buy a home, my credit rating is tarnished, and I'm going to wish I would have hunkered down.

THERAPIST: So, you don't regret things. [capturing the essence of the client's message] Worry helps you to avoid regret. [linking the message with the positive motives underlying worry]

CLIENT: Yeah. Or if I worry about it now and the outcome is still negative 10 years from now, at least I can say "I did the best I could." I thought about it. I tried to be prepared for it. And still things were out of my control . . . but at least I tried.

THERAPIST: So, you can sleep at night . . . in a way. [importantly reflecting "So, you can sleep" was *not* intended as strategic but rather, consistent with the MI spirit, is a statement that emerged from an

intent to be empathic; i.e., it's a concise restatement, and deepening, of what the client expressed]

CLIENT: Well, sleep at night (*laughing*) . . . not really. [Change talk
emerges]

THERAPIST: So, that's kind of curious. So, on the one hand, it's a way of
helping you to try to relax . . . [noticing an emergent discrepancy
between the positive intent of the worry and its actual impact;
draws the client's attention to this by reflecting it and inviting the
client to respond]

CLIENT: But it's not working! [further change talk; importantly here
the client is articulating the change talk, not the therapist]

THERAPIST: What do you make of that? So, it's designed to help you
relax. So you don't have to worry about things in the future . . . so
you don't regret stuff . . . so you don't make mistakes or fall asleep
at the switch . . . so that your life is better . . . [inviting the client
to further explore the emergent discrepancy]

CLIENT: Yeah . . . or it goes the way I want it to go down the road.
Like, I have goals for myself. And if I don't do certain things now,
I'm not going to get to where I want to be.

THERAPIST: Right. And how's that working out? [further invitation to
explore the discrepancy between the positive reasons for worry
and the outcome; importantly, this is *not* to point something
out to the client that the therapist understands—i.e., "I told you
so"—but rather to help the client explore for himself the value of
worry]

CLIENT: It's not. Nothing I'm doing seems to be working. I know this
is where I want to be, but anything in between now and then can
happen. And me worrying about that is not getting me anywhere.
All I need to do is do my best every day. [change talk] (*pause*) But I
can't turn that worry voice off. [clear statement of ambivalence—
considering the two sides together]

THERAPIST: Right. It's still difficult to do it, but you're saying that
that's something you should think about—a change in philosophy
. . . [double-sided reflection capturing both sides of the ambiva-
lence]

CLIENT: . . . is needed?

THERAPIST: Yeah. Is that right? Because you can't control things, you
need to say "I'm doing the best I can" and let go of that. [The
therapist is *not* inviting or pressuring the client to "agree" with
the therapist's statement but rather inviting him to try it on and

check the therapist's summary against his own experience; i.e., the therapist is making it clear that this is not a suggestion that comes from her—that a change in philosophy is required—but rather a further invitation to explore what has just emerged.]

CLIENT: (*looking hesitant*)

THERAPIST: But there's a voice that comes up that says "I can't do that." [double-sided reflection capturing the new emergent change voice and the anxious voice]

CLIENT: Yeah. That's exactly it. I say "I'm doing the best I can, screw off." But then that voice says "Don't kid yourself. Do you think Donald Trump ever threw his hands up and said 'Oh, I'm just trying hard'?"

THERAPIST: Absolutely. So, this voice criticizes you. It threatens you. [not pushing emerging change voice since the nonchange voice seems more alive to the client in this moment and thus continuing to reflect the change position will likely lead to resistance to the therapist]

CLIENT: Yeah . . . Do you think they were quitters? Nobody likes a quitter.

THERAPIST: So, it says, "You're going to be on skid row . . . " [not intended as finding drawbacks to the anxiety—e.g., it's critical, threatening—but rather intended in the spirit of "no wonder, that's quite a threat that you definitely would want to avoid, and worry helps you to avert such disaster"—and this is what the therapist is thinking about saying next—but, of course, it depends on where the client goes]

CLIENT: That could happen, though!

THERAPIST: Yeah, this is what it's saying to you, eh? Who knows whether it's real or not but . . .

CLIENT: It's not even letting me regain control. [emergent change talk; again the client, and not the therapist, critiques the status quo, the anxious position]

THERAPIST: There's a sense in which the sanity in you says "I know there's a different way to be, and I've felt that and I like that . . . " [The therapist aborts what she was thinking about saying and switches to what is now most alive for the client in this moment—articulating reasons to change.]

CLIENT: . . . and it's okay. [more change talk]

THERAPIST: And it's okay. And the world doesn't collapse! (*laughing*) . . . I'm guessing . . . maybe it does . . . [The therapist attempts to deepen the change talk and waits to see whether the client accepts or rejects the invitation—prepared to go to whichever side the client lands on in this moment. Here, the therapist is likely a little too eager or far ahead of the client—pushing too hard to elaborate very fledgling change talk—and likely would have been better off more gently encouraging elaboration such as "And you have a sense somehow that it might be okay. Can you say more about that?"]

CLIENT: (*laughing in response*) Not always. I'm here. I'm alive.

THERAPIST: Okay. And "I'd like to have more of that." But then this other part of you . . . the anxiety, the worry says "You're going to be unreliable, unsuccessful, you'll make mistakes . . . " [The therapist is working to bring the two sides of ambivalence together.]

CLIENT: Yeah, "Don't kid yourself or don't let yourself get off easy by saying you know this isn't really important" . . . taking the easy way out. [The client lands on the side of resistance to change talk; the therapist has placed the client back in the position of arguing for the status quo—likely by her overeager attempt to elicit further change talk.]

THERAPIST: Right. Somehow it's weak, it's easy, it's taking the easy way out. And these are all very pejorative kinds of things. It says "If you don't worry, you're going to be a good-for-nothing." [The therapist reflects what is most alive for the client in this moment.]

CLIENT: "End up like the rest of them" . . . and who the heck is the rest of them? I don't even know what that means, but it's a lie, I believe.

THERAPIST: Yeah . . . bad things will happen . . .

CLIENT: I know, it's silly . . . it's stupid . . .

THERAPIST: It doesn't sound silly. [Note that this is not a reflection. The therapist is sharing her more compassionate view of the client—is prizing—to encourage a nonpunitive understanding by the client of his own struggle.]

CLIENT: But I can't get it under control . . . I can't stop believing the lies, and it's cyclical.

THERAPIST: It's very powerful, eh? It makes a lot of sense to me that you would be struggling with this. Because even though *you* see that there is a different way of being that you might want to play around with . . . that's a pretty powerful voice, and these are pretty powerful things on the line. Like, who wants to say "Oh, well, then I just won't be successful. I'll just make mistakes"? [validation of resistance to change, link to common humanity—attempting to soften self-criticism for resisting change]

CLIENT: (*sarcastically*) Go on welfare . . . it's not important.

THERAPIST: (*sarcastically in response*) . . . "I'll just be unreliable and unprepared . . . and I don't care about that." So, there's this sense that giving up the worry would mean giving up a lot of these good things . . . the hope of being successful . . . [succinct statement of fear of change; validating positive intent of worry to reduce fear]

CLIENT: . . . is all gone . . . All of it is garbage . . .

THERAPIST: . . . if you don't worry.

CLIENT: Yeah.

THERAPIST: Worry is an important way of feeling successful . . . [validating, reframing resistance to change]

CLIENT: . . . and in control, and I'm aware of where I stand, and I'm monitoring my progress within my goals. (*pause*) But the other half of me is sitting here knowing it's a big lie. [change talk; again beginning to critically examine the value of the worry—for himself]

THERAPIST: Oh.

CLIENT: (*stated forcefully*) Yes, because it doesn't matter what life was meant to be, I don't want *my life* going on to the point where I don't enjoy anything anymore . . . [change talk again emerging but stronger; the therapist notices this shift and moves with the client in an effort to capture what is most alive now in an effort to strengthen emergent change talk]

THERAPIST: Oh, I see. So, it might work on some level . . . but on another level it's hurting you. [double-sided reflection ending with change talk since this is now more alive in the moment; since change talk is fledgling, the therapist is careful to not overstate it]

CLIENT: Yeah. It's hurting a lot. [The client responds by further elaborating change talk.]

THERAPIST: In what ways is it hurting? Can you say more about that? [elaborating change talk; again notice that a stronger statement to strengthen change talk—e.g., "And it has to go!"—would likely have yielded resistance and put the client back in the position of advocating for the status quo]

CLIENT: Well, because nothing is fun anymore. The feeling of . . . let's say I was the only one that remembered to bring that piece of paper to the meeting . . . and maybe my boss might be making note of that. I'm prepared.

THERAPIST: And that's a good thing.

CLIENT: It doesn't matter. It's so not worth it. If I forget that paper or even if I'm the only one to bring it and I feel like a shining star, I don't even allow myself to enjoy that feeling anymore. [change talk]

THERAPIST: Right. So, you're saying the rewards that it gives you to worry . . .

CLIENT: Aren't even satisfying anymore. [change talk]

THERAPIST: They are meager, compared to what you're putting in. [Reflecting change talk invites the client to elaborate.]

CLIENT: Or, when I was, like, "Okay, come this age, I want to have this type of job that I have now." When I obtained that goal, it was so fleeting . . . the reward. It was, like, "Oh yes, good for me, I got there, I worked really hard and I worried and I got everything I needed and I scored at the interviews." But now, I didn't know that this job is a nightmare. [change talk]

THERAPIST: I see . . . it just doesn't end.

CLIENT: No. I was happy for like 4 days into the training, and then I was like "*What?*"

THERAPIST: So, one of the things that the worry promises is that you'll be happy. [highlighting the discrepancy with the valued good of happiness]

CLIENT: They're lies. [change talk]

THERAPIST: Once you get there, you won't have to worry anymore.

CLIENT: It'll be a new life. And it never is, and it's just usually more troublesome . . . [change talk]

THERAPIST: . . . and more worry. It sounds like it's gotten worse, not better. [guessing at further disadvantages to the status quo; developing the discrepancy with underlying values]

CLIENT: That's true. It's a lie. Why is this happening? . . . Let's fix it and change it. [much stronger change talk and emerging commitment language]

THERAPIST: There's a sense that you want to be past this . . . you want to change this. It's selling you up the river.

CLIENT: It's invaded every part of my life. Even the things that I should be able to say "You know what? That was a huge accomplishment to get this job!" But the lie comes in and says, "You're just kidding yourself again. You got this whole job, but it brought a whole suitcase of extra worries, extra stresses, extra feeling of no turning back now." *(pause)* I'd love to have a job at a coffee shop just pouring coffee . . . and I don't mean that disrespectfully to anyone. [more change talk]

THERAPIST: You want to relax.

CLIENT: Yeah. I'd like to just check out.

THERAPIST: And that's the *real* you talking, it sounds like. [highlighting values, authentically valued directions and how the worry interferes with these]

CLIENT: That's the me that would probably be happy. If I didn't have to worry. If I could talk to people, pour them coffee, "How's your day?" get to know the regulars, move to a small town.

THERAPIST: Yes. If the real you could answer the worry, what would it say? [Increasing awareness of emerging values and practice at countering the worry by speaking from the true self and valued directions; not a bad question and invitation, but probably delivered too soon, i.e., change talk feels stronger but still quite fragile and fledgling. The therapist would likely have been better off with a more gentle prompt to encourage further elaboration of values such as "Those are the things that are more consistent with the real you. Not all this chasing your tail around trying to be super-successful," or simply "That is more of what you really want. Can you say more?"]

CLIENT: The real down-to-earth me? I would tell it to "Shut up—you're just embarrassing me!"

THERAPIST: "You're humiliating me!"

CLIENT: And I can say "What are you even worrying about A, B, and C for?" And I know that, but I believe the lie and I continue to feed it. I do things I know I shouldn't. [Ambivalence reemerges, as does frustration and self-criticism about being ambivalent.]

THERAPIST: Because it's promising important things. [validating, softening intropunitive response, i.e., "No wonder . . . "]

CLIENT: But it never delivers. Or it has . . . but how come it delivers but it doesn't let me feel the significance of getting there? Why does it take that away? [Change talk reemerges.]

THERAPIST: So, it kind of gives you something on the one hand and then takes it away with the other.

CLIENT: Yeah, that happened with work. I wonder what else that has happened with. [change talk]

THERAPIST: That's happened a lot, it sounds like. [gently inviting the client to elaborate change talk]

CLIENT: 'cause I'm never happy. I could win the lottery, and the lie would be like "You're still nothing, get rid of that money, donate it" . . . just anything to make me not enjoy.

THERAPIST: Right, I see. [The client accepts the invitation and the therapist invites the client to further elaborate the emerging change position.] And how much does that fit with what you really want in life? If you were to think about what it is you really want life to be like . . . I'm sure it wouldn't be like this. [increasing awareness of values and discrepancy between worry and values]

CLIENT: No.

THERAPIST: What would you want it to be like?

CLIENT: Normal.

THERAPIST: What does that mean?

CLIENT: Someone that can sleep at night, someone that isn't pushing other people away, someone that isn't always annoyed or . . . feeling on that tip of "I'm going snap at the littlest thing." I'd like to be in control, calm, stop sighing. I'd like to function on a more reasonable level. To be able to blend in and then be able to do those things with no regrets . . . no "I should haves" or "What if's." And know the boundary of "Does this matter or does it not matter?" . . . or "What's important and what's not?" Because the worry . . . the lie . . . tells me it's important to worry, because "Look, you did get that job, you did get the car," . . .

THERAPIST: So, you want all these things, and the worry tries to convince you that it helped you to get them.

CLIENT: But the new additional liar that I seem to have put together by talking about this with you is not even letting me enjoy it. It's taking it away. [more change talk; importantly, this emerges from the client's own critical evaluation based on the new awareness of what the worry was originally intended to help with and promote—meeting core needs]

THERAPIST: It never lets you rest. [continuing to invite the client to elaborate change talk by reflecting]

CLIENT: No. It's never done.

THERAPIST: And you can't think of many instances, if any, where the promised land has come into view.

CLIENT: Been greener . . . right. Like, on my list to do is to start traveling. Now that I've got the car and everything is in my stupid schedule. So, I start traveling and the voice comes on and it's, like, "Yeah, well, okay now, you're in so much debt, your net value, and blah, blah, blah . . ."

THERAPIST: It's never a good time.

CLIENT: No. And then it's made it so not fun that now it's just a checkmark on my list.

THERAPIST: Right. And it's almost incompatible with fun. [continuing to develop discrepancy; guessing at another downside of the worry]

CLIENT: Yeah!

THERAPIST: As long as the worry is there, you can't get what you really want in life.

CLIENT: How do we fix this, 'cause that's it [reemerging commitment language]

THERAPIST: That's something you're really wanting to look at.

CLIENT: I want to enjoy what I'm working for.

THERAPIST: Yeah, this has cost you a lot.

CLIENT: But now that I know . . . I don't know it all, but just by talking here I'm kinda seeing that it's all a lie . . . but then there's a solution too. There's a way to fix this. [strong commitment language, indicating a need to shift to helping the client envision and begin experimenting with taking action]

THERAPIST: Yes, absolutely. So, maybe that's a good place to leave it for today and see what comes up, if anything. [evocatively encouraging the client to reflect for himself about possible solutions]

CLIENT: Okay. Yeah, that would be good to just kind of reflect.

THERAPIST: So, how did you feel about our session today? Things you did and did not like . . . [The therapist is checking her own perception of how well she was understanding, matching client needs, etc., and prepared to revise as needed to better match the client's needs.]

CLIENT: I feel a bit better.

THERAPIST: [Here, the therapist could have asked for more specifics as a guide to revising the intervention style to ensure responsivity to this individual client's needs.] So, if you were to sort of summarize what you got out of talking together today . . . [Rather than the therapist summarizing, the client is evocatively asked to summarize.]

CLIENT: It's bigger than I even thought, and it pushes . . . the worrying and anxiety pushes me to try to get to places, but it's the places that I get to . . . the worry penetrates and that voice comes on and tells I'm lying. So, I need to figure out why that is happening, and then I can fix it. I didn't even think of that. I just thought I don't enjoy life anymore. I never connected that it's because that voice and the anxiety and the worry are being lugged around on my shoulders everywhere I go . . . even if I'm getting there . . . where I want to be, I still carry that monkey. So, understanding that is major. [This summary was much more accurate to the client's experience than what the therapist could have offered; further it helps consolidate his growing interest and commitment to change.]

In this exchange, there was a palpable shift in Frank's view of the value of worrying and an emergent increase in the desirability and importance of change. The increased change talk over the course of the interaction had a very emergent quality and indicated that Frank himself, rather than the therapist, had assessed the value of his worry and decided it "was not worth it"; that is, the client, and not the therapist, was in the position of deciding about change and articulated the reasons, desires, and need to change. The role of the therapist was extremely important in helping him consider his dilemma and the seductiveness of the worry. The therapist's role consisted of reflecting on, empathically following, elaborating, and validating Frank's struggle and the positive motives underlying his worry. Through this process, Frank could see his dilemma and ambivalence more clearly and then decide what *he* wanted to do about it. Accordingly, the client articulated having a "new understanding" of his situation.

Importantly here, cultivating and retaining the spirit of MI seemed critical in order that the discrepancies were developed not for the purpose of correcting the client or pointing out "the error of his ways" but rather to enable him to see the merits of change (through this own expert position). The therapist does not have an apriori agenda or goal to "get the client to see" that he is misguided or wrong to worry. Rather, the stance and intent are exploratory and discovery-oriented, where the therapist brings significant curiosity to the task of understanding the client, in the service of helping him to better understand himself—both the motives or the functions driving the "problem" (worry and related behavior, in this instance) and his incentives for and views on change.

When this is done consistently and well, the client is then in a position of greater self-understanding and arguably greater self-compassion and can then begin to evaluate the degree to which the anxiety or worry is an ally or an obstacle to helping him to reach important goals or enact important values in his life (e.g., "I now see that by worrying I am trying to relax, but is this behavior helping or hurting my efforts to relax? . . . moving me toward or away from this important goal?"). The client then begins to question or critically challenge the anxious behavior and his assumptions. And since the problematic assumptions and behaviors to which they give rise are typically inconsistent with innate valued goals, the client moves toward expressing greater change talk (e.g., reasons, need, and desires to change).

To further underscore the importance of MI spirit in helping the client explore ambivalence, flexible movement (and course correction) by the therapist is continually required as the dialogue proceeds, in order to capture shifts in what is most alive and emergent for the client. That is, it is impossible to know or plan in advance what the right thing is to say at any moment since it must be responsive to the immediate (and continually changing) context of "moving with the client." For example, early in the exploration the therapist finds herself genuinely articulating that "worry is an important way of being successful." Here, in working to reframe resistance to change (as positive rather than negative), the therapist almost appears to be an advocate for worry—or at least is on the side of worry, since that is the position the client is occupying at that time. Again, the therapist is not asserting a position that "worry is a fabulous thing" but rather is consistently validating and resonating with the positive underlying motives and intentions behind the worry (attempting to be prizing and affirming). Later in the exploration, the therapist inhabits exactly the opposite position, saying and genuinely meaning that "as long as worry is there, you can't get what you really want" (i.e., worry is not a key to success, but actually thwarts this goal). In order to maintain MI spirit, the therapist engages in the often difficult task of working hard to bracket their own perspective on the issue of the usefulness or harmfulness of worry, in order to remain open and responsive to exploring and expanding the client's own views and understanding in each moment.

Frank also exhibited multiple markers of increased readiness for change such as increasing change talk (e.g., "It's not even letting me regain control," "It's hurting a lot"), beginning to actively ponder solutions and expressing commitment language ("There's a way to fix this, too") and reduced ambivalence (i.e., becoming quicker to challenge the advantages of the status quo with change talk). Thus, during subsequent sessions, the therapist continued to watch for such signs of readiness in order to gauge whether a shift was needed toward helping him conceptualize an action plan.

In the next session, Frank began to exhibit further markers of readiness for change, including taking steps to change. For example, he described his anxiety as "not as alive" as earlier and said he was starting to "talk back to it." For example:

CLIENT: Doing the old thinking makes me feel worse. When I go against it I feel better. I need to keep going with this and keep making healthier choices. [change talk; commitment language]

THERAPIST: You're not buying it as much anymore. You can separate yourself from it a bit better.

CLIENT: Yeah. I don't feel as drawn into it.

THERAPIST: It's like it's not the absolute truth anymore. You're starting to object to it. You're starting to say, "Well, I don't know that I agree." And you want to keep building on that. That's important. [supporting the client's shift to developing and envisioning further steps to change]

Frank also described that he was beginning to entertain thoughts about quitting his job, shifting career direction, and going back to school to work toward a job that gave him greater enjoyment and satisfaction (i.e., actively considering change). He described his job as a major obstacle in his efforts to move forward with change since it was a major source of anxiety and worry, and he asked to put this matter on the agenda to work on in the session (to which the therapist responded, reinforcing his autonomy, "Absolutely. You're the boss"). He also began to express more acceptance and compassion toward himself. For example, he noted that for the first time he was entertaining the idea that "life can get tricky, and it's okay to say that." That is, he had been idealistic as a young person, but it's okay and healthy to recognize if a job is not a good fit with what one desires in life and to admit that one is "not invincible." Rather than wishing to persevere in an untenable and unhealthy work situation, he expressed greater interest in exploring what type of job would be a better fit for him, given his emerging values stressing greater self-nurturance and self-care, health, and happiness.

As soon as Frank's priority to reevaluate his job situation arose, the therapist worked to help him understand his ambivalence about this in the context of continuing to increase awareness of his values and strengthening self-efficacy and commitment to change. For example:

THERAPIST: Why is it okay to think about switching jobs? [consolidating commitment to change]

CLIENT: Because I want to touch base with myself more. Be real with it. Deal with it instead of putting a wall up and saying "Put your head down and go."

THERAPIST: You're tired of playing by the old rules. It's driven you to places . . . [change talk]

CLIENT: . . . that aren't pretty . . .

THERAPIST: . . . and aren't you. And you can get in touch with what you really want. And that's okay. [bringing in client values to help further consolidate commitment to change]

CLIENT: It's okay.

THERAPIST: It doesn't mean that you're weak.

CLIENT: Yeah! Like I'm starting to see that I need to allow myself time and space to think about positive things . . . to get better . . . look after myself more. [change talk; increasing resolve for change]

THERAPIST: And that sounds huge for you.

CLIENT: That's huge! That is so important. To say "You've learnt this, and now what can you do to change it?" And be good to myself about it, versus being "Oh, be tough . . . suck it up." That got so far out of control. Because I have that mentality on everything. [increasing commitment to change]

THERAPIST: That driven workhorse life is about suffering and sucking it up. So, getting better, being less worried, less depressed, is really important. And worth sacrificing for. And you seem to need to make some changes to get there. [reflecting commitment language]

CLIENT: And it's not always comfortable. Like it took me the whole week to verbalize that I'm going to prepare myself to look for another job.

THERAPIST: Wow. A whole week! (*laughing*) [trying to soften high self-expectations that change should be rapid or easy]

CLIENT: (*laughing in response*) It's not a long time . . .

THERAPIST: But you're saying it won't always be comfortable to change, but you need to give yourself time, be patient with yourself, expect it to be uncomfortable. [actively helping the client prepare for change]

DEVELOPING AN ACTION PLAN AND EXPERIMENTING WITH CHANGE

Frank was clearly wishing to further consider taking action toward change and was continuing to push for and prepare for this. To match the approach to the client's stage of readiness, I shifted to an action-oriented CBT approach aimed at helping Frank conceptualize and experiment with implementing change in his worrying. However, the spirit and methods of MI—in particular, the core skills of empathic reflection; creating an atmosphere of discovery and experimentation; drawing on and evoking the client's ideas and resources in pursuing change; supporting client autonomy while contributing therapist ideas or expertise on change; continually being sensitive to the client's receptivity to change efforts, level of engagement, and any reemergent ambivalence; and rolling with resistance as needed to help process such fluctuations in motivation for change—continued to infuse and inform my efforts despite the movement away from building motivation for change to supporting taking action to change.

In introducing the rationale for using CBT to manage Frank's worry, I was attuned to his receptivity to this throughout and explicitly inquired about his reactions at multiple points in the discussion. That is, when infusing MI into psychoeducation or skills training, the therapist takes care not to "lose" the client by presenting ideas didactically and clearly communicates that the two can proceed only if the information is judged by the client as potentially useful (continuing with permission). Through Frank's nonverbal responses (attentive listening, head nodding, smiling, etc.) as well as his explicit statements that he was eager to learn practical strategies for responding to and reducing worry, we continued. Frank was provided with some readings on identifying maladaptive thoughts, and I suggested that he closely monitor his worry episodes.

In the next session, Frank came in with a binder containing the reading materials and completed self-monitoring sheets. He reported:

CLIENT: When I read some of those materials, I realized that my bottom lines or self rules are way out to lunch . . . When I repeat them back to myself, it sounds so ridiculous. I would never say that to a friend of mine. [clearly engaged with making effort to change]

THERAPIST: So, you're saying that you need to start talking to yourself in healthier ways. Did you have a specific example of an unhealthy bottom line?

CLIENT: "You have between the ages of 30 and 40 to excel in a career. That's it." I just kept repeating it to myself and I thought, "That is probably the stupidest thing I've ever said to myself." [increased ability to distance self from previous anxious thinking style; clearly on the side of wanting to change, and therapist needs to support this movement]

THERAPIST: It seems so off the mark. So untrue. What seems inaccurate about it? [elaborating change talk and strengthening the alternative, nonanxious, perspective]

CLIENT: Well, it's just not true. You need to have successes and nonsuccesses in your career, and it doesn't matter at what age they happen.

THERAPIST: And I'm not sure if this part of it is for you, but it also seems like so much pressure! [Socratic questioning in an MI style, to further elaborate new nonanxious responding]

CLIENT: Yeah. It's so unnecessary. It doesn't mean you'll die or something if you're not a VP by 40. Like what . . . live the remaining 50 years of my life under the bed.

THERAPIST: And maybe another thing worth looking at is to ask "What does it mean to excel, anyway?" Career success is just one way to excel, but there are other parts to life. Like your anxiety is making this all or nothing. If you don't excel in your career, and in this little window of time, all is lost. [Socratic questioning in an MI style]

CLIENT: Yeah. You know, I just absorbed that idea from a friend who said, "If you don't excel in your career by 40, you're screwed." But it's not really me, not what I want.

THERAPIST: So, this is a good example of identifying what you say to yourself now . . . becoming more aware of that . . . and how you could respond differently that is more balanced. And it might be a good idea if we continue to work on developing healthier responses to the worry. Would you agree?

CLIENT: Yeah. Because I also thought, "If that is just one of them, I really want to look at my bottom lines." Like, I'd like to make a list. I really want to look at those and say "Yes" or "No" or "Maybe this needs to be a bit modified." My rules of life are off-kilter, and that is creating all kinds of problems.

THERAPIST: That sounds like a good idea. In fact, today I could introduce you to a specific strategy for helping with that, called the Thought Record. Would that make sense to show you that today? [asking permission to provide advice]

CLIENT: Yes. That sounds good. I also find that my thoughts are pretty buried and it takes some time to uncover them.

THERAPIST: Absolutely. That's an important observation, and the Thought Record should help you with that.

Here I worked within the action CBT phase by using empathy to help the client further access, understand, elaborate, and strengthen the emerging alternative, nonanxious perspective. Again, the greater attention to process that comes with training in MI is important in conducting CBT. Here, I continuously attempt to attune to where the client is in the process of change and work to assess and provide what is needed in that moment, with continual preparedness to back off or move forward more quickly, depending on the client's responses (i.e., rolling with resistance).

Even within the action phase, rather than requiring the client to be where the therapist is, the therapist can go where the client is and bring in specific strategies, tools, and methods to help the client with the goals they have identified. In this process, there is also an absence of "I told you so" (i.e., discovering what the therapist already knew, or therapist-as-expert), but rather a context of self-discovery by the client—in this case, one of needing to respond more effectively to anxious thinking. If Frank did not express this explicitly, then I could easily have suggested this (while explicitly preserving client autonomy) and gauge his receptivity and response to this suggestion in order to determine direction. With Frank's stated interest in developing nonanxious responses to anxious thoughts, I also began to bring in Socratic questions to help him strengthen the nonaxious perspective (e.g., "And what does it mean to excel, anyway?"). Again, consistent with the spirit of MI, it is both the timing of the introduction of these methods (introducing them in a tentative way that preserves autonomy) and their attunement to the client's response (engagement or resistance) that guide the therapist and determine whether he or she will persist with these methods or not.

Working with CBT methods, I then helped Frank apply and generalize this new perspective to specific examples of worry and anxiety triggers as they unfolded in Frank's life. At this point, I introduced other specific CBT methods to assist him with this task, such as relaxation training and deep breathing, to facilitate a soothing response to threat and worry triggers. Psychoeducation about the process of change was also introduced. For example:

> "It is common for the old anxious perspective to try to squeeze out the new perspective, and it can do so easily because it is so well practiced. So, that is normal, and you can expect that to happen. Do not be surprised when it does. People can often get discouraged or frustrated that, because they see a different way of being and responding in one situation, it doesn't automatically happen all the time. It's important to recognize that this takes practice and work. And we want you to be triggered, because this gives you important opportunities to work through these situations and apply the new perspective and tools. So, it can be useful to have you monitor your worry and anxiety and then bring some of these examples in to our sessions so we can put our heads together to help support you in making these changes that are important to you. How does that sound?"

PROCESSING ACTION STEPS
TO DEVELOP SELF-EFFICACY

Later in therapy (about the fourth or fifth session), Frank came in reporting a significant drop in his anxiety and worry level (down to 30 out of 100). I saw this as a further opportunity to develop and support Frank's self-efficacy by processing these change efforts in a client-centered manner. A spirit of curiosity was brought to this in helping Frank explore and become more aware of effective anxiety management strategies for him. I also used psychoeducation to reinforce the normalcy and validity of Frank's experience.

THERAPIST: If you are willing, can you say what you are doing differently that is making you less anxious?

CLIENT: I lost an account on Friday, but I wasn't anxious about it. I remembered what we were talking about last week [the therapist provided the client with a worksheet for capturing and describing anxious predictions, on the one hand, and actual outcomes, on the other], you know, "What do I think is going to happen, and what is probably going to happen?" And I thought, "You're going to get fired and never get another job." But then I thought, "You're probably not going to get fired, and even if you did you have the tools to pick up the pieces—should that happen, you're not screwed."

THERAPIST: So, it sounds like you didn't automatically buy the anxious prediction. You stepped back and entertained a more reasonable alternative.

CLIENT: Yeah. And Sundays are difficult days for me, and I heard this voice, "You should be worried, because you'll have to deal with your boss on Monday" . . . My inner self was saying that. And I thought "No." Because, as soon as I started to entertain the idea of becoming anxious and worrying I started to feel anxious, and I just said "Whoa—stop right there!" That was such a difference.

THERAPIST: So, if I hear you right, you're thinking that the thoughts that pop into your mind may be just thoughts. And you can choose to engage with them or not. [empathic reflection]

CLIENT: Yeah. I thought, "It's Sunday . . . It's *my* time . . . I don't have to think about work today. It's okay to not be anxious." And it really worked this time, but I would like to keep going with that and test that out more . . . it seems to make sense.

THERAPIST: That's something you feel you need to continue. You need to keep testing these thoughts. And it sounds like you are finding that it's possible to look at the original situation to see if it's really as bad or threatening as the anxiety tells you it is. [empathic reflection; building on change talk] And for what it's worth, in my experience, I would have to say that I agree with you that practice is important; working with this new way of thinking so that that new voice eventually becomes the automatic one versus the threat voice. [providing psychoeducation with autonomy]

ROLLING WITH RESISTANCE IN THE ACTION PHASE

Using empathic reflection and cognitive methods, we worked through specific situations from Frank's self-monitoring that were worry-inducing for him, including work-related situations, worry about family members, and social interactions. Moreover, I rolled with resistance (although it was minimal) throughout the therapy whenever it occurred. For example:

CLIENT: Sometimes I worry that telling myself "Nothing is going to happen, relax" is going too far. When does it become too much?

THERAPIST: You're concerned that if you take this relaxation thing too far, you might become lazy, unproductive. [empathic reflection to clarify underlying belief; rolling with resistance]

CLIENT: Yeah, like I might not want to do anything.

THERAPIST: So, I could be wrong about this, but that sounds like the anxious voice—"Watch out, you could take this too far . . . it could backfire on you . . . you were deluding yourself by thinking this would make you happy . . . in fact, it could make you unhappy." It's trying to warn you . . . to protect you somehow. Only you can really know where the truth lies and what's best. What do you think? [reframing and rolling with resistance; eliciting client expertise]

CLIENT: Actually, I've been so much happier by working on being less worried.

THERAPIST: And have you collapsed? become lazy? [Again, this is asked not for the purpose of persuading the client to relinquish the anxious belief but rather to help him explore the accuracy of the belief himself so that he can decide whether to retain it or not.]

CLIENT: Actually, no. I still know when I need to plug in and do stuff.

THERAPIST: So, there's a risk with making this change . . . turning off the worry more. But the anxiety also seems to magnify that risk.

If you think about it, the chances are pretty low that allowing
yourself to be more relaxed will turn you into a lazy, irrespon-
sible person who doesn't care about anything. That's just not you.
[empathic reflection]
CLIENT: That's true. I am very responsible . . . too responsible, actually.

Or, consider another example of moving back to MI to navigate
ambivalence temporarily during the action phase. Here, we were discussing
something he was noticing and disliked in his manner with others.

CLIENT: I find myself complaining a lot . . . being really negative . . .
especially about past criticisms of others of my performance . . . I
hate it and I want to stop it. I just carry those old encounters with
me. I don't let go of them.

THERAPIST: What have you tried to stop it?

CLIENT: I remind myself to stop and remind myself that it doesn't help,
but I see myself just going ahead and do it anyway. It's really frus-
trating.

THERAPIST: Absolutely. You know you don't want to do it, but you
do it anyway. So, there is something important about doing this
somehow. [exploring the motives that perpetuate the behavior,
good things about the "problem"]

CLIENT: Yes, but it seems so stupid and useless.

THERAPIST: Well, this may seem like a weird question, but "What is
appealing about complaining?" It seems to be serving some purpose. [understanding and reframing resistance]

CLIENT: (pause) It feels good.

THERAPIST: Because . . .

CLIENT: . . . because it's not true.

THERAPIST: So, this is a kind of protest . . . a type of self-defense.
"You can't say that about me—it's not true!" A kind of setting the
record straight. [reframing complaining as reflecting an underlying positive motive]

CLIENT: It's like, I want to hear that somehow, and I want others to
hear it too.

THERAPIST: Absolutely. [i.e., validation—"Naturally you would want
to hear that"] And it feels good to remind yourself and others that
you're not like that . . . "it's not true what you said about me. Only
I can know the truth about myself!" [empathically resonating]

CLIENT: I really believe that. I like that a lot. [emergent change talk]

THERAPIST: And it sounds like you are tired of giving other people the power to say what is true about you.

CLIENT: Absolutely. It's wrong. [change talk]

THERAPIST: If you were to speak from that part of you that you've discovered more recently . . . the one that responds differently . . . what would you say? [seeking to elaborate change position]

CLIENT: It's really coming from them. They need to be critical, put others down, in order to make themselves feel better, superior. [change talk]

THERAPIST: So, it's not necessarily a reflection on you. [empathic listening]

CLIENT: Right. And even if there was some truth to it, I can accept that. Like when I have to train new staff. I really work hard to challenge them in a constructive way. I don't attack them. I think there is no place for that, but at the same time I don't just praise them all the time if I know they're capable of better work. [change talk]

THERAPIST: So, there's a way of being constructively critical . . . of helping people grow rather than deflating them . . . and you value that. [empathic listening; elaborating values]

CLIENT: (*pause*) I guess I need to do that for myself. [change talk]

THERAPIST: What do you mean?

CLIENT: I need to respond to myself in a way that doesn't take unconstructive criticism seriously . . . doesn't give it more credibility than it deserves. [change talk]

THERAPIST: So, more congruence . . . more authenticity . . . consistency with what you really want to stand for. It's kind of striking actually that you don't value others attacking people so that they can feel superior, yet you find yourself falling into that same trap in a way, in complaining about others. [developing discrepancy]

CLIENT: Yikes! You're absolutely right. I need to be more myself, model to myself what I believe. [change talk]

Here, I temporarily shifted back to MI (rolling with resistance, elaborating good things about the current problematic response) in the context of markers of "stuckness." Here, I was able to move in more quickly to evoke an alternative response, given the strong therapeutic alliance and history of productive collaborative work. Frank is also able to more quickly access a more adaptive alternative response, given the work that has been occurring on strengthening these responses. In general, rather than "supplying the answers," the therapist seeks to evoke them from the client, is careful to not "push" for change, and remains attuned to signs of resistance, indicating a greater need to shift to more MI. I suggested a possible homework task that Frank could try if he was interested. With his permission to proceed with the suggestion, I suggested that he spend some time dialoguing with the hurt part of himself to soothe and heal these old wounds by allowing his new perspective to respond to these old wounds. Frank seemed (and indicated) that he was quite receptive to attempting this.

BUILDING ON AND ENCOURAGING FURTHER ACTION

Following this, I then introduced the rationale for exposure work, and Frank was receptive to monitoring safety behaviors in order to work on reducing them. The safety behaviors Frank identified included checking (e.g., frequent phone calls to his mother), reassurance seeking (e.g., regarding his job performance), avoiding worry triggers (e.g., answering and returning work-related phone calls), and distractions (e.g., watching television). Frank was receptive to the rationale for exposure, and subsequently he actively engaged with these exercises, resulting in significant benefits.

I then introduced the rationale for worry exposure and invited Frank to consider conducting an in-session worry exposure exercise, such as visualizing being stuck in a sales job endlessly, performing poorly, not achieving, or being repeatedly reprimanded by his boss—and being chronically miserable as a result. After working through some initial reluctance (using strategies for rolling with resistance), helping him weigh the pros and cons, and reinforcing that it was ultimately his decision, Frank attempted this with success in promoting habituation and further decentering from worrisome thoughts. We also spent some time on relapse prevention, including anticipating and working through possible catastrophic reactions to possible future triggers.

Frank's score on a measure of worry (the Penn State Worry Questionnaire) after 10 sessions of therapy was 22, a score at the 10th percentile, compared to population norms (Gillis, Haaga, & Ford, 1995), and a reduction of over 6 standard deviations from his score before treatment. Moreover, his scores on measures of depression, anxiety, and stress (the Depression Anxiety Stress Scale; Lovibond & Lovibond, 1995) were all in the normal range posttreatment. He described himself as "a lot more laid back," "more normal," "able to sleep now," and "in control of my emotions and not run by anxiety."

HELPFUL ELEMENTS OF THERAPY
FROM FRANK'S PERSPECTIVE

Toward the end of therapy, I ask my clients to provide their feedback on helpful and unhelpful aspects of therapy, how they experienced the process of therapy, and what they identify as key contributors to their change efforts. This feedback mainly provides me with information to help refine my developing theory on how change comes about and what processes in therapy positively and negatively influence this process. In terms of the process of therapy, Frank remarked that the first few sessions (i.e., the MI) were "so powerful" and evoked "huge lightbulb moments." He noted that a lot of these moments occurred through empathic reflection. For example, he stated:

> "When you would sort of reiterate what I just said but maybe even just change the intonation or just sort of ask me what I just said . . . 'Does that make sense?' or 'Tell me about that . . . how you feel.' And as I would get talking through it I'd start to think, 'Oh! I get it.'"

Frank also noted that it was very helpful for him to think about the genesis of his anxiety, that is, Where did he get these beliefs? He noted that his anxious thinking derived from his father's voice of "Do better, be better, worry about this . . . take care of it now." And this discovery allowed him to feel more hopeful and confident about being able to change. He reported subsequently feeling "Okay, then I can handle this!" and "This is going to be a lot . . . not easier . . . but not as scary to change as I thought." In short, Frank reported experiencing the MI as helpful in encouraging him to be more open to considering change and increasing his confidence in being able to change.

In considering later sessions, Frank remarked that he liked how the therapy was more practical and was "structured but flexible," in that if something more important arose he could put that on the agenda. Frank also noted that understanding his bottom lines (i.e., core beliefs), "looking at things in perspective . . . like what's the worst that could happen, and is that really that bad?," and "Understanding that my bottom lines were unrealistic" were very helpful for him. Frank also confirmed that initially he was skeptical about being able to benefit from therapy, since he thought it was going to involve "telling me I shouldn't think of things that negatively and everything is just a basket of kittens." When he had this initial impression of therapy, Frank thought he could not engage with this task, as it didn't appear credible to him. Frank noted, however, that therapy was very different from his initial expectations. For example, he stated

"But it wasn't about that, it was about *my* idea of things and how my life should operate within *my own rules* for myself. And I really got the sense that 'Okay; it does not have to be this way. It's your choice if you want to continue." Even though you never said it like that, that's what I got . . . like, you're giving me the tools and it's up to me what I want to do with them.' "

That is, Frank's observations on his experience highlighted the importance of developing awareness of the motives underlying his worry; the therapist's use of empathic reflection to help him develop this awareness; improved readiness and confidence about change; therapist flexibility and client-centeredness; assistance with helping him critically examine his underlying beliefs; and the therapist communicating and reinforcing his autonomy and self-determination throughout all stages of the therapy process. In terms of the focus of this book, Frank valued initial work on building his motivation for change and the therapist's infusion of MI spirit and methods—especially preservation of his autonomy—during the action phase, when helping him to take steps toward change.

EPILOGUE

∝

Training and Future Directions

LEARNING MOTIVATIONAL INTERVIEWING

MI appears deceptively simple, yet it is not easy to do. Concepts such as empathy, unconditional regard, prizing clients when they oppose you or the direction of therapy, and related ideas can all appear straightforward on the surface but are very difficult to implement in practice. For me, learning MI has been the most challenging (and rewarding) aspect of my professional experience to date.

Integrating more and less directive approaches, as described and outlined in this book, is particularly challenging. The seamless movement between promoting acceptance and facilitating action is especially difficult for those experienced with more structured action-oriented methods and is among the most formidable challenges to using MI effectively. One can realize the limits of exhortation for change but still struggle to let go of these methods in the moment. Despite these challenges, MI does appear to be complementary and compatible with other methods of working with clients suffering from anxiety and related problems.

As Miller and Rollnick (2009) note, MI involves a complex set of skills that are used flexibly, responding to moment-to-moment changes in the client. A common metaphor for capturing the process of MI is dancing rather than wrestling with clients. Dancing well and in harmony with another requires a continual and high level of attunement and responsivity to one's partner—noticing moment-to-moment fluctuations in order to know what to do next. It is also akin to the process of learning to play a musical instrument—and then learning to play in harmony with another.

Clinicians should resist the temptation to assume they already do MI, since self-perceived competence in MI and in reflective listening more generally can be unrelated to actual observed proficiency (Miller & Mount, 2001). Clinicians should also avoid assuming that adequate MI proficiency can be attained by simply attending a workshop (Miller, Yahne, Moyers, Martinez, & Pirritano, 2004)—much as one cannot learn to play the violin over lunch (Miller & Rollnick, 2009). Rather, MI is a complex clinical skill that is developed and refined over a long period of time, which is particularly true since MI is more a way of being with clients, or an attitude, than it is a particular set of techniques.

Some guidance on additional readings and resources for learning more about MI is provided in the Appendix. While this is a good place to start, *ideally* seeking out training and feedback from a practitioner competent in MI best facilitates effective implementation of MI skills.[1] Miller and colleagues' work on training in MI suggests that direct coaching and feedback are important to competent MI practice (e.g., Miller et al., 2004). That is, as with any complex skill, one can only learn so much by reading about it or even watching competent practitioners. Rather, integrating these skills into your practice will gradually provide you with a readily available source of feedback and experience. Although there are currently few trainers who specialize in the application of MI to anxiety, there are many MI trainers who are proficient in the core skills of MI. In addition, developing a peer support group in your particular setting or locale can be useful in listening to one another's practice and providing peer support and consultation.

In training others in MI, I have also discovered that critically reviewing videotape is invaluable. There is a tremendous amount to be learned from watching even brief samples of videotape. If you have an MI trainer, or someone who is more proficient in MI than you are currently, this is a valuable exercise to integrate in acquiring feedback. But even in the absence of this, listening carefully to your own videotapes or audiotapes of sessions can be extremely useful. When doing so, you might stop the tape frequently and brainstorm other possible empathic reflections, ways of rolling with resistance, ways of responding to change talk, and the like. Such practice is especially helpful, in my experience, since these are complex responses that take time to generate. They are a product of multiple steps (hearing what the client is trying to say, selecting something to focus on, then putting that into words to formulate and deliver). Students learning empathy and other foundational MI skills often bemoan, "If only I could hit 'pause' after a client statement." If you tape a few sessions, you can actually create

---

[1] See *www.motivationalinterview.org* for a list of MI trainers, training events, and training exercises.

that space to brainstorm and refine MI-consistent responses. So, much like practicing a tennis swing outside of the context of an actual game, practice with videotape (yours or even others') makes it more likely that such responses will come more easily in actual therapy sessions. Moreover, such practice also helps you to develop facility in learning to inhabit the frame of reference of the client (to imagine what he or she might be sensing, feeling, or thinking)—a critical first step in communicating empathy.

FUTURE DIRECTIONS

The extension of MI to the treatment of anxiety and related problems such as depression is quite recent. Research on MI for anxiety and depression is in the early stages, and the existing findings are generally quite promising (Westra, Aviram, & Doell, 2011). However, clearly, well-controlled research trials are needed to adequately evaluate the recommendations offered in this book. This is especially important, given that MI is being widely recommended by clinical researchers for inclusion in existing treatments for many major mental health problems, and yet very few well-controlled studies have been conducted to date. We also need research to identify whom MI works for and why MI works (i.e., what particular elements of MI are responsible for its positive effects). That is, we need process research that uncovers both helpful and hindering therapist responses and ways of being, on a moment-to-moment basis, during therapy sessions (both within MI itself and when MI spirit and methods are being integrated with other therapies). Such research will not only advance our understanding of effective ways of enhancing motivation and client engagement in the therapy process, but it will also facilitate training.

Although much research remains to be conducted, MI makes good clinical sense. Arguably, as clinicians we struggle routinely with issues of client motivation and nonadherence. In part, this reflects the nature of change, which is highly turbulent and fraught with uncertainty, conflict, fear, and ambiguity. Thus, having a way of being that facilitates working through the dilemmas that often stall or derail movement toward change represents a welcome and significant clinical advancement. Such skills are an important addition to any therapist's clinical arsenal. And, as I have suggested in this book, the spirit underlying MI (and the accompanying methods) do not have to be abandoned when clients move toward taking action to change.

Moreover, many of the skills within MI (as detailed in this book in work with anxiety and related problems) are important components of effective clinical practice more generally and enjoy strong empirical support. Thus, honing skills such as providing empathy, building self-efficacy, working with rather than against resistance, and facilitating the client's active involvement in the process of therapy are arguably an important part of any effective clinical practice. I hope you will evaluate the methods outlined in this book for yourself, however, and in the context of your own practice—since only you can determine whether these recommendations truly have merit.

APPENDIX

❧

Resources and Recommended Readings

MOTIVATIONAL INTERVIEWING WEBSITE

The MI website (*www.motivationalinterview.org*) has reference material, training DVDs, a list of MI trainers and training events, a bibliography of research on MI, and other useful links.

BOOKS

Arkowitz, H., Westra, H. A., Miller, W. R., & Rollnick, S. (Eds.). (2008). *Motivational interviewing in the treatment of psychological problems*. New York: Guilford Press.

Bohart, A. C., & Greenberg, L. S. (Eds.). (1997). *Empathy reconsidered: New directions in psychotherapy*. Washington, DC: American Psychological Association.

Bohart, A. C., & Tallman, K. (2003). *How clients make therapy work: The process of active self-healing*. Washington, DC: American Psychological Association.

Engle, D., & Arkowitz, H. (2006). *Ambivalence in psychotherapy: Facilitating readiness to change*. New York: Guilford Press.

Miller, W. R., & Rollnick, S. (2002). *Motivational interviewing: Preparing people for change* (2nd ed.). New York: Guilford Press.

Miller, W. R., & Rollnick, S. (in press). *Motivational interviewing: Helping people change* (3rd ed.). New York: Guilford Press.

Naar-King, S., & Suarez, M. (2011). *Motivational interviewing with adolescents and young adults*. New York: Guilford Press.

Rogers, C. R. (1951). *Client-centered therapy*. Boston: Houghton Mifflin.

Rogers, C. R. (1965). *Client-centered therapy: Its current practice, implications, and theory.* Boston: Houghton Mifflin.

Rogers, C. R. (1980). *A way of being.* Boston: Houghton Mifflin.

Rollnick, S., Miller, W. R., & Butler, C. C. (2008). *Motivational interviewing in health care: Helping patients change behavior.* New York: Guilford Press.

Rosengren, D. B. (2009). *Building motivational interviewing skills: A practitioner workbook.* New York: Guilford Press.

Sheldon, K. M., Williams, G., & Joiner, T. (2003). *Self-determination theory in the clinic: Motivating physical and mental health.* New Haven, CT: Yale University Press.

ARTICLES AND CHAPTERS

Arkowitz, H., & Westra, H. (2004). Integrating motivational interviewing and cognitive behavior therapy in the treatment of depression and anxiety. *Journal of Cognitive Psychotherapy, 18,* 337–350.

Arkowitz, H., & Westra, H. A. (Guest Ed.). (2009). *Journal of Clinical Psychology: In Session, 65.*—Special issue on MI and psychotherapy. Includes articles on MI for anxiety, depression, social anxiety, spousal abuse, suicidality, and drinking during pregnancy.

Burns, D. D., & Auerbach, A. (1996). Therapeutic empathy in cognitive-behavioral therapy: Does it really make a difference? In P. M. Salkovskis (Ed.), *Frontiers of cognitive therapy* (pp. 135–164). New York: Guilford Press.

McKay, D., & Bouman, T. K. (2008). Enhancing cognitive-behavioral therapy for monosymptomatic hypochondriasis with motivational interviewing: Three case illustrations. *Journal of Cognitive Psychotherapy, 22,* 154–166.

Rogers, C. R. (1957) The necessary and sufficient conditions of therapeutic personality change. *Journal of Consulting Psychology, 21,* 95–103.

Rogers, C. R. (1975). Empathic: An unappreciated way of being. *The Counseling Psychologist, 5,* 2–10.

Watson, J. C. (2001). Re-visioning empathy. In D. J. Cain & J. Seerman (Eds.), *Humanistic psychotherapies: Handbook of research and practice* (pp. 445–472). Washington, DC: American Psychological Association.

Watson, J. C., Goldman, R., & Vanderschot, G. (1998). Empathic: A postmodern way of being. In L. S. Greenberg, J. C. Watson, & G. Lietaer (Eds.), *Handbook of experiential psychotherapy* (pp. 61–81). New York: Guilford Press.

Westra, H. A. (2004). Managing resistance in cognitive behavioural therapy: application of motivational interviewing in mixed anxiety depression. *Cognitive Behaviour Therapy, 33,* 161–175.

Westra, H. A., & Arkowitz, H. (2010). Combining motivational interviewing and cognitive-behavioral therapy to increase treatment efficacy for generalized anxiety disorder. In D. Sookman & R. L. Leahy (Eds.), *Treatment resistant anxiety disorders: Resolving impasses to symptom remission* (pp. 199–232). New York: Routledge.

Westra, H. A., & Arkowitz, H. (Guest Ed.). (2011). *Cognitive and Behavioral*

Practice, 18.—Special issue on integrating MI with CBT for a range of mental health problems. Includes articles on MI for eating disorders, suicidal ideation, OCD, GAD, depression, and substance abuse.

Westra, H. A., & Phoenix, E. (2003). Motivational enhancement therapy in two cases of anxiety disorder: New responses to treatment refractoriness. *Clinical Case Studies, 2,* 306–322.

References

Ahmed, M., & Westra, H. A. (2009). Impact of a treatment rationale on expectancy and engagement in cognitive behavioral therapy for social anxiety. *Cognitive Therapy and Research, 33*, 314–322.

Ahmed, M., Westra, H. A., & Constantino, M. J. (2010). *Interpersonal process during resistance in CBT associated with high versus low client outcome expectations: A micro-process analysis.* Paper presented at the annual meeting of the Society for Psychotherapy Research, Pacific Grove, CA.

Alexander, F., & French, T. M. (1946). *Psychoanalytic therapy: Principles and application.* New York: Ronald Press.

Amrhein, P. C., Miller, W. R., Yahne, C. E., Palmer, M., & Fulcher, L. (2003). Client commitment language during motivational interviewing. *Journal of Consulting and Clinical Psychology, 71*, 862–878.

Angus, L. E., & Kagan, F. (2009). Therapist empathy and client anxiety reduction in motivational interviewing: "She carries with me, the experience." *Journal of Clinical Psychology, 65*, 1156–1167.

Arkowitz, H., & Burke, B. (2008). Motivational interviewing as an integrative framework for the treatment of depression. In H. Arkowitz, H. A. Westra, W. R. Miller, & S. Rollnick (Eds.), *Motivational interviewing in the treatment of psychological problems* (pp. 145–173). New York: Guilford Press.

Arkowitz, H., & Westra, H. A. (2004). Integrating motivational interviewing and cognitive behavioral therapy in the treatment of depression and anxiety. *Journal of Cognitive Psychotherapy, 18*(4), 337–350.

Aspland, H., Llewelyn, S., Hardy, G. E., Barkham, M., & Stiles, W. (2008). Alliance ruptures and rupture resolution in cognitive-behavior therapy: A preliminary task analysis. *Psychotherapy Research, 18*, 699–710.

Aviram, A., & Westra, H. A. (2011). The impact of motivational interviewing on resistance in cognitive behavioral therapy for generalized anxiety disorder. *Psychotherapy Research, 21*(6), 698–708.

Barlow, D. H. (2002). *Anxiety and its disorders: The nature and treatment of anxiety and panic* (2nd ed.). New York: Guilford Press.

Beech, C., & Brazier, D. (1995). Empathy for a real world. In R. Hutterer, G. Pawlowsky, P. Schmid, & R. Stipsits (Eds.), *Client centered and experiential therapy: A paradigm in motion*. Vienna: Lang.

Benjamin, L. S. (2003). Interpersonal reconstructive therapy: An integrative, personality-based treatment for complex cases. New York: Guilford.

Beutler, L. E., Harwood, T. M., Michelson, A., Song, X., & Holman, J. (2011). Resistance/Reactance level. *Journal of Clinical Psychology, 67*, 133–142.

Beutler, L. E., Moleiro, C. M., & Talebi, H. (2002a). Resistance in psychotherapy: What conclusions are supported by research. *Journal of Clinical Psychology, 58*, 207–217.

Beutler, L. E., Moleiro, C. M., & Talebi, H. (2002b). Resistance. In J. Norcross (Ed.), *Psychotherapy relationships that work: Therapist contributions and responsiveness to patients* (pp. 129–144). Oxford, UK: Oxford University Press.

Binder, J. L., & Strupp, H. H. (1997). "Negative process": A recurrently discovered and underestimated facet of therapeutic process and outcome in the individual psychotherapy of adults. *Clinical Psychology: Science and Practice, 4*, 121–139.

Bohart, A. C., & Greenberg, L. S. (Eds.). (1997). *Empathy reconsidered: New directions in psychotherapy*. Washington, DC: American Psychological Association.

Bohart, A. C., Elliott, R. E., Greenberg, L. S., & Watson, J. C. (2002). Empathy. In J. Norcross (Ed.), *Psychotherapy relationships that work: Therapist contributions and responsiveness to patients* (pp. 89–108). Oxford, UK: Oxford University Press.

Bohart, A. C., & Tallman, K. (1999). *How clients make therapy work*. Washington, DC: American Psychological Association.

Borkovec, T. D. (1994). The nature, functions, and origins of worry. In G. C. L. Davey & F. Tallis (Eds.), *Worrying: Perspectives on theory, assessment, and treatment* (pp. 5–34). New York: Wiley.

Borkovec, T. D., Newman, M. G., Pincus, A. L., & Lytle, R. (2002). A component analysis of cognitive-behavioral therapy for generalized anxiety disorder and the role of interpersonal problems. *Journal of Consulting and Clinical Psychology, 70*, 288–298.

Borkovec, T. D., & Roemer, L. (1995). Perceived functions of worry among generalized anxiety disorder subjects: Distraction from more emotionally distressing topics? *Journal of Behavior Therapy and Experimental Psychiatry, 26*, 25–30.

Bozarth, J. (1990). The essence of client centered therapy. In G. Lietaer, J. Rombauts, & R. Van Balen (Eds.), *Client-centered and experiential psychotherapy in the nineties* (pp. 59–64). Leuven, Belgium: Leuven University Press.

Britton, P. C., Patrick, H., Wenzel, A., & Williams, G. C. (2011). Integrating motivational interviewing and self-determination theory with cognitive behavioral therapy to prevent suicide. *Cognitive and Behavioral Practice, 18*, 16–27.

Britton, P. C., Williams, G. C., & Connor, K. R. (2008). Self-determination theory, motivational interviewing, and the treatment of clients with acute suicidal ideation. *Journal of Clinical Psychology, 64*, 52–66.

Brody, A. E. (2009). Motivational interviewing with a depressed adolescent. *Journal of Clinical Psychology, 65,* 1168—1179.

Brody, A. E., Arkowitz, H., & Allen, J. J. B. (2008). *Development and validation of a self-report measure of ambivalence toward change.* Poster presented at the annual meeting of the Association for Psychological Science, Chicago.

Brown, T. A., & Barlow, D. H. (2009). A proposal for a dimensional classification system based on the sheared features of the DSM-IV anxiety and mood disorders: Implications for assessment and treatment. *Psychological Assessment, 21,* 256–271.

Brown, T. A., Campbell, L. A., Lehman, C. L., Grisham, J. R., & Mancill, R. B. (2001). Current and lifetime comorbidity of the DSM-IV anxiety and mood disorders in a large clinical sample. *Journal of Abnormal Psychology, 110,* 49–58.

Buckner, J. D. (2009). Motivation enhancement therapy can increase utilization of cognitive-behavioral therapy: The case of social anxiety disorder. *Journal of Clinical Psychology, 65,* 1195–1206.

Buckner, J. D., Roth Ledley, D., Heimberg, R. G., & Schmidt, N. B. (2008). Treating comorbid social anxiety and alcohol use disorders: Combining motivation enhancement therapy with cognitive behavioral therapy. *Clinical Case Studies, 7,* 208–223.

Burke, B. L., Arkowitz, H., & Menchola, M. (2003). The efficacy of motivational interviewing: A meta-analysis of controlled clinical trials. *Journal of Consulting and Clinical Psychology, 71,* 843–861.

Burns, D. D. (2006). *When panic attacks: The new drug-free anxiety therapy that can change your life.* New York: Morgan Road Books.

Burns, D. D., & Auerbach, A. (1996). Therapeutic empathy in cognitive-behavioral therapy: Does it really make a difference? In P. M. Salkovskis (Ed.), *Frontiers of cognitive therapy* (pp. 135–164). New York: Guilford Press.

Burns, D. D., & Nolen-Hoeksema, S. (1991). Coping styles, homework compliance and the effectiveness of cognitive-behavioral therapy. *Journal of Consulting and Clinical Psychology, 59,* 305–311.

Burns, D. D., & Nolen-Hoeksema, S. (1992). Therapeutic empathy and recovery from depression in cognitive-behavioral therapy: A structural equation model. *Journal of Consulting and Clinical Psychology, 60,* 441–449.

Burns, D. D., Shaw, B. F., & Crocker, W. (1987). Thinking styles and coping strategies of depressed women: An empirical investigation. *Behaviour Research and Therapy, 25*(3), 223–225.

Burns, D. D., & Spangler, D. (2000). Does psychotherapy homework lead to changes in depression in cognitive behavioral therapy? Or does clinical improvement lead to homework compliance? *Journal of Consulting and Clinical Psychology, 68,* 46–59.

Burns, D. B., Westra, H. A., & Trockel, M. (2010). *Motivation and rapid changes in depression in two inpatient samples.* Manuscript submitted for publication.

Cassidy, J., & Shaver, P. R. (Eds.) (2008). *Handbook of attachment: Theory, research, and clinical applications* (2nd ed.). New York: Guilford Press.

Castonguay, L. G., Goldfried, M. R., Wiser, S., Raue, P. J., & Hayes, A. M. (1996). Predicting the effect of cognitive therapy for depression: A study of unique and common factors. *Journal of Consulting and Clinical Psychology, 64,* 497–504.

Catanzaro, S. J., & Mearns, J. (1999). Mood-related expectancy, emotional experience and coping behavior. In I. Kirsch (Ed.), *How expectancies shape experience* (pp. 67–92). Washington, DC: American Psychological Association.

Chamberlain, P., Davis, J. P., Forgatch, M., Frey, J., Patterson, G. R., Ray, J., et al. (1985). *The Therapy Process Code: A multidimensional system for observing therapist and client interactions.* Unpublished coding manual.

Chamberlain, P., Patterson, G. R., Reid, J. B., Kavanagh, K., & Forgatch, M. S. (1984). Observation of Client Resistance. *Behavior Therapy, 15,* 144–155.

Christiana, J. M., Gilman, S. E., Guardino, M., Mickelson, K., Morselli, P. L., Olfson, M., et al. (2000). Duration between onset and time of obtaining initial treatment among people with anxiety and mood disorders: An international survey of members of mental health patient advocate groups. *Psychological Medicine, 30,* 693–703.

Cole, D. A., Peeke, L. G., Martin, J. M., Truglio, R., & Seroczynski, A. D. (1998). A longitudinal look at the relation between depression and anxiety in children and adolescents. *Journal of Consulting and Clinical Psychology, 66,* 451–460.

Collins, K. A., Westra, H. A., Dozois, D. J. A., & Burns, D. D. (2004). Gaps in accessing treatment for anxiety and depression: Challenges for the delivery of care. *Clinical Psychology Review, 24,* 583–616.

The COMBINE Study Research Group (2003). Testing combined pharmacotherapies and behavioral interventions in alcohol dependence (The COMBINE Study): A pilot feasibility. *Alcoholism: Clinical and Experimental Research, 27,* 1123–1131.

Constantino, M. J., Arnkoff, D. B., Glass, C. R., Ametrano, R. M., & Smith, J. Z. (2011). Expectations. *Journal of Clinical Psychology, 67,* 184–192.

Constantino, M. J., Arnow, B. A., Blasey, C., & Agras, W. S. (2005). The association between patient characteristics and the therapeutic alliance in cognitive-behavioral and interpersonal therapy for bulimia nervosa. *Journal of Consulting and Clinical Psychology, 73,* 203–211.

Constantino, M. J., Castonguay, L. G., & Schut, A. J. (2002). The working alliance: A flagship for the "scientist-practitioner" model in psychotherapy. In G. S. Tryon (Ed.), *Counseling based on process research: Applying what we know* (pp. 81–131). Boston: Allyn & Bacon.

Deci, E. L., & Ryan, R. M. (1985). *Intrinsic motivation and self-determination in human behavior.* New York: Plenum.

de Haan, E., Oppen, P., Van Balkom, A. J. L. M., Spinhoven, P., Hoogduin, K. A. L., & Van Dyck, R. (1997). Prediction of outcome and early vs. late improvement in OCD patients treated with cognitive behaviour therapy and pharmacotherapy. *Acta Psychiatrica Scandinavica, 96,* 354–361.

Devilly, G. J., & Borkovec, T. D. (2000). Psychometric properties of the Credibility/Expectancy Questionnaire. *Journal of Behavior Therapy and Experimental Psychiatry, 31,* 73–86.

Dowd, E. T., Milne, C. R., & Wise, S. L. (1991). The Therapeutic Reactance Scale:

A measure of psychological reactance. *Journal of Counseling and Development*, 69, 541–545.

Dozois, D. J. A., & Westra, H. A. (2004). The nature of anxiety and depression: Implications for prevention. In D. J. A. Dozois & K. S. Dobson (Eds.), *The prevention of anxiety and depression: Theory, research and practice* (pp. 9–41). Washington, DC: American Psychological Association.

Dozois, D. J. A., Westra, H. A., Collins, K. A., Fung, T. S., & Garry, J. K. F. (2004). Stages of change in anxiety: Psychometric properties of the University of Rohde Island Change Assessment (URICA) Scale. *Behaviour Research and Therapy*, 42, 711–729.

Duncan, B. L., Hubble, M. A., & Miller, S. D. (1997). *Psychotherapy with impossible cases: The efficient treatment of therapy veterans*. New York: Norton.

Ellard, K. K., Fairholme, C. P., Boisseau, C. L., Farchione, T. J., & Barlow, D. H. (2010). Unified protocol for the transdiagnostic treatment of emotional disorders: Protocol development and initial outcome data. *Cognitive and Behavioral Practice*, 17, 88–101.

Engle, D. E., & Arkowitz, H. (2006). *Ambivalence in psychotherapy: Facilitating readiness to change*. New York: Guilford Press.

Festinger, L. (1957). *A theory of cognitive dissonance*. Stanford, CA: Stanford University Press.

Finn, S. E., & Tonsager, M. E. (1997). Information-gathering and therapeutic models of assessment: Complementary paradigms. *Psychological Assessment*, 9, 374–385.

Francis, N., Rollnick, S., McCambridge, J., Butler, C., Lane, C., & Hood, K. (2005). When smokers are resistant to change: Experimental analysis of the effect of patient resistance on practitioner behaviour. *Addiction*, 100, 1175–1182.

Geller, J., Drab-Hudson, D. L., Whisenhunt, B. L., & Srikameswaran, S. (2004). Readiness to change dietary restriction predicts outcomes in the eating disorders. *Eating Disorders*, 12, 209–224.

Geller, S. M., & Greenberg, L. S. (2002). Therapeutic presence: Therapists® experience of presence in the psychotherapy encounter. *Person Centered and Experiential Psychotherapies*, 1, 71–86.

Gilbert, P. (1993). Defence and safety: Their function in social behaviour and psychopathology. *British Journal of Clinical Psychology*, 32, 131–153.

Gilbert, P. (2005). Compassion and cruelty: A biopsychosocial approach. In P. Gilbert (Ed.), *Compassion: Conceptualizations, research, and use in psychotherapy* (pp. 9–74). New York: Routledge.

Gilbert, P. (2009). *The compassionate mind: A new approach to life's challenges*. Oakland, CA: New Harbinger.

Gilbert, P. (2010). Attachment and the importance of affection. In *Compassion focused therapy* (pp. 39–42). New York: Routledge.

Gilbert, P., & Irons, C. (2005). Focused therapies and compassionate mind training for shame and self-attacking. In P. Gilbert (Ed.), *Compassion: Conceptualizations, research, and use in psychotherapy* (pp. 263–325). New York: Routledge.

Gillis, M. M., Haaga, D. A. F., & Ford, G. T. (1995). Normative values for the Beck Anxiety Inventory, Fear Questionnaire, Penn State Worry Questionnaire, and Social Phobia and Anxiety Inventory. *Psychological Assessment, 7,* 450–455.

Greenberg, L. S. (2002). *Emotion-focused therapy: Coaching clients to work through their feelings.* Washington, DC: American Psychological Association.

Greenberg, L. S., Rice, L. N., & Elliott, R. (1993). *Facilitating emotional change: The moment-by-moment process.* New York: Guilford Press.

Greenberg, L. S., Elliott, R., Watson, J. C., & Bohart, A. C. (2001). Empathy. *Psychotherapy, 38,* 380–384.

Greenberg, R. P., Constantino, M. J., & Bruce, N. (2005). Are patient expectations still relevant for psychotherapy process and outcome? *Clinical Psychology Review, 26,* 657–678.

Greenberger, D., & Padesky, C. A. (1995). *Mind over mood: A cognitive therapy treatment manual for clients.* New York: Guilford Press.

Hayes, S. C., Strosahl, K. D., & Wilson, K. G. (2012). *Acceptance and commitment therapy: The process and practice of mindful change* (2nd ed.). New York: Guilford Press.

Helbig, S., & Fehm, L. (2004). Problems with homework in CBT: Rare exception or rather frequent? *Behavioral and Cognitive Psychotherapy, 32*(3), 291–301.

Hettema, J., Steele, J., & Miller, W. R. (2005). Motivational interviewing. *Annual Review of Clinical Psychology, 1*(1), 91–111.

Huppert, J. D., Bufka, L. F., Barlow, D. H., Gorman, J. M., Shear, M. K., & Woods, S. W. (2001). Therapists, therapist variables, and cognitive behavioral therapy outcome in a multicenter trial for panic disorder. *Journal of Consulting and Clinical Psychology, 69,* 747–755.

Jobes, D. A., & Mann, R. E. (1999). Reasons for living versus reasons for dying: Examining the internal debate of suicide. *Suicide and Life-Threatening Behavior, 29*(2), 97–104.

Jungbluth, N. J., & Shirk, S. R. (2009). Therapist strategies for building involvement in cognitive-behavioral therapy for adolescent depression. *Journal of Consulting and Clinical Psychology, 77,* 1179–1184.

Kampman, M., Keijsers, G. P. J., Hoogduin, C. A. L., & Hendriks, G. J. (2008). Outcome prediction of cognitive behaviour therapy for panic disorder: Initial symptom severity is predictive for treatment outcome, comorbid anxiety or depressive disorder, cluster C personality disorders and initial motivation are not. *Behavioural and Cognitive Psychotherapy, 36,* 99–112.

Kazantzis, N., Lampropoulos, G. K., & Deane, F. P. (2005). A national survey of practicing psychologists' use and attitudes toward homework in psychotherapy. *Journal of Consulting and Clinical Psychology, 73*(4), 742–748.

Keijsers, G. P. J., Hoogduin, C. A. L., & Schaap, C. P. D. R. (1994a). Prognostic factors in the behavioral treatment of panic disorder with and without agoraphobia. *Behavior Therapy, 25,* 689–708.

Keijsers, G. P. J., Hoogduin, C. A. L., & Schapp, C. P. D. R. (1994b). Predictors of treatment outcome in the behavioural treatment of obsessive–compulsive disorder. *British Journal of Psychiatry, 165,* 781–786.

Keijsers, G. P. J., Kampman, M., & Hoogduin, C. A. L. (2001). Dropout prediction in cognitive behavior therapy for panic disorder. *Behavior Therapy, 32,* 739–749.

Keijsers, G. P. J., Schaap, C. P. D. R., Hoogduin, C. A. L., Hoogsteyns, B., & de Kemp, E. C. M. (1999). Preliminary results of a new instrument to assess patient motivation for treatment in cognitive-behavior therapy. *Behavioural and Cognitive Psychotherapy, 27,* 165–179.

Kertes, A., Westra, H. A., & Aviram, A. (2010). *Therapist effects in cognitive behavioral therapy: Client perspectives.* Paper presented at the annual meeting of the Society for Psychotherapy Reserach, Pacific Grove, CA.

Kessler, R. C., McGonagle, K. A., Zhao, S., Nelson, C. B., Hughes, M., Eshleman, S., et al. (1994). Lifetime and 12-month prevalence of DSM-III-R psychiatric disorders in the United States: Results from the National Comorbidity Survey. *Archives of General Psychiatry, 51,* 8–19.

Kiesler, D. J. (1996). *Contemporary interpersonal theory research: Personality, psychopathology, and psychotherapy.* New York: Wiley.

Kirsch, I. (1990). *Changing expectations: A key to effective psychotherapy.* Pacific Grove, CA: Brooks/Cole.

Kovacs, M., & Beck, A. T. (1977). The wish to die and the wish to live in attempted suicides. *Journal of Clinical Psychology, 33*(2), 361–365.

Kushner, M. G., & Sher, K. J. (1989). Fear of psychological treatment and its relation to mental health service avoidance. *Professional Psychology: Research and Practice, 20,* 251–257.

Kushner, M. G., & Sher, K. J. (1991). The relation of treatment fearfulness and psychological service utilization: An overview. *Professional Psychology: Research and Practice, 22,* 196–203.

Leahy, R. L. (2001). *Overcoming resistance in cognitive therapy.* New York: Guilford Press.

Linehan, M. M. (1997). Validation and psychotherapy. In L. S. Greenberg & A. C. Bohart (Eds.), *Empathy reconsidered: New directions in psychotherapy* (pp. 353–392). Washington, DC: American Psychological Association.

Littell, J. H., & Girvin, H. (2002). Stages of change: A critique. *Behavior Modification, 26,* 223–273.

Lovibond, P. F., & Lovibond, S. H. (1995). The structure of negative emotional states: Comparison of the Depression Anxiety Stress Scales (DASS) with the Beck Depression and Anxiety Inventories. *Behaviour Research and Therapy, 33,* 335–343.

Mahoney, M. J. (2003). The experience of change. In *Constructive psychotherapy* (pp. 70–192). New York: Guilford Press.

Marcus, M., Westra, H. A., Angus, L., & Kertes, A. (2011). Client experiences of Motivational Interviewing for Generalized Anxiety Disorder, *Psychotherapy Research, 21*(4), 447–461.

Martell, C. R., Addis, M. E., & Jacobson, N. S. (2001). *Depression in context: Strategies for guided action.* New York: Norton.

Martin, D. G. (1999). *Counseling and therapy skills* (2nd ed.). Long Grove, IL: Waveland Press.

McCabe, R. E., Rowa, K., Antony, M. M., Young, L., & Swinson, R. P. (2008).

Using motivational enhancement to augment treatment outcome following exposure and response prevention for obsessive compulsive disorder: Preliminary findings. Paper presented at the Annual Meeting of the Association for Behavioral and Cognitive Therapies, Orlando, FL.

McConnaughy, E. A., Prochaska, J. O., & Velicer, W. F. (1983). Stages of change in psychotherapy: Measurement and sample profiles. *Psychotherapy: Theory, Research, and Practice, 20,* 368–375.

McHugh, M. D. (2007). Readiness for change and short-term outcomes of female adolescents in residential treatment for anorexia nervosa. *International Journal of Eating Disorders, 40,* 602–612.

McKay, D., & Bouman, T. K. (2008). Enhancing cognitive-behavioral therapy for monosymptomatic hypochondriasis with motivational interviewing: Three case illustrations. *Journal of Cognitive Psychotherapy, 22,* 154–166.

Mendlowicz, M. V., & Stein, M. B. (2000). Quality of life in individuals with anxiety disorders. *American Journal of Psychiatry, 157,* 669–682.

Miller, W. R., Benefield, R. G., & Tonigan, J. S. (1993). Enhancing motivation for change in problem drinking: A controlled comparison of two therapist styles. *Journal of Consulting and Clinical Psychology, 61,* 455–461.

Miller, W. R., Hedrick, K. E., & Orlofsky, D. R. (1991). The Helpful Responses Questionnaire: A procedure for measuring therapeutic empathy. *Journal of Clinical Psychology, 47,* 444–448.

Miller, W. R., & Johnson, W. R. (2008). A natural language screening measure for motivaton to change. *Addictive Behaviors, 33,* 1177–1182.

Miller, W. R., & Mount, K. A. (2001). A small study of training in motivational interviewing: Does one workshop change clinician and client behavior? *Behavioural and Cognitive Psychotherapy, 29,* 457–471.

Miller, W. R., & Rollnick, S. (2002). *Motivational interviewing: Preparing people for change* (2nd ed.). New York: Guilford Press.

Miller, W. R., & Rollnick, S. (2009). Ten things that motivational interviewing is not. *Behavioural and Cognitive Psychotherapy, 37,* 129–140.

Miller, W. R., & Rollnick, S. (in press). *Motivational interviewing: Helping people change* (3rd ed.). New York: Guilford Press.

Miller, W. R., & Rose, G. S. (2009). Toward a theory of motivational interviewing. *American Psychologist, 64,* 527–537.

Miller, W. R., Yahne, C. E., Moyers, T. B., Martinez, J., & Pirritano, M. (2004). A randomized trial of methods to help clinicians learn motivational interviewing. *Journal of Consulting and Clinical Psychology, 71,* 754–763.

Moyers, T. B., Martin, T., Manuel, J. K., & Miller, W. R. (2003). *The Motivational Interviewing Treatment Integrity (MITI) code* (coding manual). Albuquerque, NM: University of New Mexico, Center on Alcoholism, Substance Abuse and Addictions.

Moyers, T. B., Martin, T., Manuel, J. K., Hendrickson, S. M. L., & Miller, W. R. (2005). Assessing competence in the use of motivational interviewing. *Journal of Substance Abuse Treatment, 28,* 19–26.

Moyers, T. B., & Rollnick, S. (2002). A motivational interviewing perspective on resistance in psychotherapy. *Journal of Clinical Psychology, 58*(2), 185–193.

Murphy, R. T. (2008). Enhancing combat veterans' motivation to change posttraumatic stress disorder symptoms and other problem behaviors. In H. Arkowitz, H. A. Westra, W. R. Miller, & S. Rollnick (Eds.), *Motivational interviewing in the treatment of psychological problems* (pp. 57–84). New York: Guilford Press.

National Institute of Clinical Excellence (2004). *Clinical guidelines for the management of anxiety.* Retrieved December 1, 2009, from *www.nice.org.uk/Guidance/CG.*

Neimeyer, R. A., Kazantzis, N., Kassler, D. M., Baker, K. D., & Fletcher, R. (2008). Group cognitive behavioral therapy for depression outcomes predicted by willingness to engage in homework, compliance with homework, and cognitive restructuring skills. *Cognitive Behaviour Therapy, 37,* 199–215.

Newman, C. F. (1994). Understanding client resistance: Methods for enhancing motivation for change. *Cognitive and Behavioral Practice, 1,* 47–69.

Norton, P. J., & Hope, D. A. (2005). Preliminary evaluation of a broad-spectrum cognitive-behavioral group therapy for anxiety. *Journal of Behavior Therapy and Experimental Psychiatry, 36,* 79–97.

Norton, P. J., & Price, E. C. (2007). A meta-analytic review of adult cognitive-behavioral treatment outcome across the anxiety disorders. *Journal of Nervous and Mental Disease, 195*(6), 521–531.

O'Hare, T. (1996). Readiness for change: Variation by intensity and domain of client distress. *Social Work Research, 20,* 13–17.

Orlinsky, D. E., Grawe, K., & Parks, B. K. (1994). Process and outcome in psychotherapy: Noch einmal. In A. E. Bergin & S. L. Garfield, (Eds.), *Handbook of psychotherapy and behavior change* (4th ed., pp. 270–376). Oxford, UK: Wiley.

Papageorgiou, C. & Wells, A. (2001). Positive beliefs about depressive rumination: Development and preliminary validation of a self-report scale. *Behaviour Therapy, 32,* 13–26.

Patterson, G. R., & Forgatch, M. S. (1985). Therapist behavior as a determinant for client noncompliance: A paradox for the behavior modifier. *Journal of Consulting and Clinical Psychology, 53,* 846–851.

Pelletier, L., Tuson, K. M., & Haddad, N. K. (1997). Client Motivation for Therapy Scale: A measure of intrinsic motivation, extrinsic motivation and amotivation for therapy. *Journal of Personality Assessment, 68,* 414–435.

Price, M., Anderson, P., Henrich, C. C., & Rothbaum, B. O. (2008). Greater expectations: Using hierarchical linear modeling to examine expectancy for treatment outcome as a predictor of treatment response. *Behavior Therapy, 39,* 398–405.

Prochaska, J. O. (1999). How do people change and how can we change to help many more people? In M. A. Hubble, B. L. Duncan, & S. D. Miller (Eds.), *The heart and soul of change* (pp. 227–255). Washington, DC: American Psychological Association.

Prochaska, J. O., & Norcross, J. C. (2004). *Systems of psychotherapy: A transtheoretical analysis* (5th ed.). New York: Wadsworth.

Purdon, C., Rowa, K., & Antony, M. M. (2004). *Treatment fears in individuals awaiting treatment of OCD.* Paper presented at the meeting of the Association for Advancement of Behavior Therapy, New Orleans, LA.

Ramnero, J., & Ost, L.-G. (2004). Prediction of outcome in the behavioural treatment of panic disorder with agoraphobia. *Cognitive Behaviour Therapy, 4,* 176–180.

Rector, N. A., Bagby, R. M., Segal, Z. V., Joffe, R. T., & Levitt, A. (2000). Self-criticism and dependency in depressed patients treatment with cognitive therapy or pharmacotherapy. *Cognitive Therapy and Research, 24,* 571–584.

Rennie, D. L. (1994). Clients' accounts of resistance in counselling: A qualitative analysis. *Canadian Journal of Counselling, 28,* 43–57.

Rhodes, R. H., Hill, C. E., Thompson, B. J., & Elliott, R. (1994). Client retrospective recall of resolved and unresolved misunderstanding events. *Journal of Counseling Psychology, 41,* 473–483.

Rogers, C. R. (1951). *Client-centered therapy.* Boston: Houghton Mifflin.

Rogers, C. R. (1956). Client-centered therapy. *Journal of Counseling Psychology, 3,* 115–120.

Rogers, C. (1957). The necessary and sufficient conditions of therapeutic personality change. *Journal of Consulting Psychology, 21,* 95–103.

Rogers, C. R. (1961). *On becoming a person.* Oxford, UK: Houghton Mifflin.

Rogers, C. R. (1965). *Client-centered therapy: Its current practice, implications, and theory.* Boston: Houghton Mifflin.

Rogers, C. R. (1975). Empathic: An unappreciated way of being. *The Counseling Psychologist, 5,* 2–10.

Rogers, C. R. (1980). *A way of being.* Boston: Houghton Mifflin.

Rogers, C. R., & Shostrom, E. (2000). *Three approaches to psychotherapy: Part 1. Carl Rogers.* Corona Del Mar, CA: Psychological & Educational Films.

Rollnick, S., & Miller, W. R. (1995). What is motivational interviewing? *Behavioural and Cognitive Psychotherapy, 23,* 325–334.

Rollnick, S., Miller, W. R., & Butler, C. C. (2008). *Motivational interviewing in health care: Helping patients change behavior.* New York: Guilford Press.

Rowa, K., Gifford, S., McCabe, R., Antony, M. M., & Purdon, C. (2010). *Treatment fears in anxiety disorders: Development and validation of the Treatment Ambivalence Questionnaire.* Manuscript submitted for publication.

Rubin, H. C., Rapaport, M. H., Levine, B., Gladsjo, J. K., Rabin, A., Auerbach, M., et al. (2000). Quality of well being in panic disorder: The assessment of psychiatric and general disability. *Journal of Affective Disorders, 57,* 217–221.

Sachse, R., & Elliott, R. (2001). Process–outcome research on humanistic therapy variables. In D. J. Cain & J. Seerman (Eds.), *Humanistic psychotherapies: Handbook of research and practice* (pp. 83–116). Washington, DC: American Psychological Association.

Safran, J. D., & Muran, J. C. (1996). The resolution of ruptures in the therapeutic alliance. *Journal of Consulting and Clinical Psychology, 64,* 447–458.

Safran, J. D., Muran, J. C., Samstag, L. W., & Stevens, C. (2002). Repairing alliance ruptures. In J. C. Norcross (Ed.), *Psychotherapy relationships that work: Therapist contributions and responsiveness to patients* (pp. 235–254). Oxford, UK: Oxford University Press.

Safren, S. A., Heimberg, R. G., & Juster, H. R. (1997). Clients' expectancies and their relationship to pretreatment symptomatology and outcome of cognitive-behavioral group treatment for social phobia. *Journal of Consulting and Clinical Psychology, 65*(4), 694–698.

Sanderson, W. C., & Bruce, T. J. (2007). Causes and management of treatment-resistant panic disorder and agoraphobia: A survey of expert therapists. *Cognitive and Behavioral Practice, 14,* 26–35.

Segal, Z. V., Williams, J. M. G., & Teasdale, J. D. (2001). *Mindfulness-based cognitive therapy for depression: A new approach to preventing relapse.* New York: Guilford Press.

Sheldon, K. M., Williams, G., & Joiner, T. (2003). *Self-determination theory in the clinic: Motivating physical and mental health.* New Haven, CT: Yale University Press.

Simon, G. E., Ludman, E. J., Tutty, S., Operskalski, B., & Von Korff, M. (2004). Telephone psychotherapy and telephone care management for primary care patients starting antidepressant treatment: A randomized controlled trial. *Journal of the American Medical Association, 292,* 935–942.

Simpson, H. B., Zuckoff, A., Page, J. R., Franklin, M. E., & Foa, E. B. (2008). Adding motivational interviewing to exposure and ritual prevention for obsessive–compulsive disorder: An open pilot trial. *Cognitive Behaviour Therapy, 37,* 38–49.

Simpson, H. B., & Zuckoff, A. (2011). Using motivational interviewing to enhance treatment outcome in people with obsessive–compulsive disorder. *Cognitive and Behavioral Practice, 18,* 28–37.

Sutton, S. (2001). Back to the drawing board?: A review of applications of the transtheoretical model to substance use. *Addiction, 96,* 175–186.

Swartz, H. A., Shear, M. K., Wren, F.J., Greeno, C., Sales, E., Sullivan, B. K., et al. (2005). Depression and anxiety among mothers who bring their children to a pediatric mental health clinic. *Psychiatric Services, 56,* 1077–1083.

Swartz, H. A., Zuckoff, A., Frank, E., Spielvogle, H. N., Shear, M. K., Fleming, M.A.D., et al. (2006). An open-label trial of enhanced brief interpersonal psychotherapy in depressed mothers whose children are receiving psychiatric treatment. *Depression and Anxiety, 23,* 398–404.

Swinson, R. P. (2006). Working group on management of anxiety disorders. Clinical practice guidelines: Management of anxiety disorders. *Canadian Journal of Psychiatry, 51,* lS–90S.

Taylor, C. (1990). *Human agency and language.* New York: Cambridge University Press.

Tolin, D. F., & Maltby, N. (2008). Motivating treatment-refusing clients with obsessive–compulsive disorder. In H. Arkowitz, H. A. Westra, W. R. Miller, & S. Rollnick (Eds.), *Motivational interviewing in the treatment of psychological problems* (pp. 85–108). New York: Guilford Press.

Treasure, J., Katzman, M., Schmidt, U., Troop, N., Todd, G., & deSilva, P. (1999). Engagement and outcome in the treatment of bulimia nervosa: First phase of a sequential design comparing motivation enhancement therapy and cognitive behavioral therapy. *Behaviour Research and Therapy, 37,* 405–418.

Van Vorrhees, B. W., Fogel, J., Pomper, B. E., Marko, M., Reid, N., Watson, N., et al. (2009). Adolescent dose and ratings of an internet-based depression prevention program: A randomized trial of primary care physician brief advice versus a motivational interview. *Journal of Cognitive and Behavioral Psychotherapies, 9*, 1–19.

Vogel, P. A., Hansen, B., Stiles, T. C., & Gotestam, K. G. (2006). Treatment motivation, treatment expectancy, and helping alliance as predictors of outcome in cognitive behavioral treatment of OCD. *Journal of Behavior Therapy and Experimental Psychiatry 37*, 247–255.

Wagner, C. C., & Ingersoll, K. S. (2008). Beyond cognition: Broadening the emotional base of motivational interviewing. *Journal of Psychotherapy Integration, 18*, 191–206.

Wampold, B. E. (2001). *The great psychotherapy debate: Models, methods, and findings.* Mahwah, NJ: Erlbaum.

Watson, J. C. (2001). Re-visioning empathy. In D. J. Cain & J. Seerman (Eds.), *Humanistic psychotherapies: Handbook of research and practice* (pp. 445–472). Washington, DC: American Psychological Association.

Watson, J. C., Goldman, R., & Vanaerschot, G. (1998). Empathic: A postmodern way of being. In L. S. Greenberg, J. C. Watson, & G. Lietaer (Eds.), *Handbook of experiential psychotherapy* (pp. 61–81). New York: Guilford Press.

Watson, J. C., & McMullen, E. J. (2005). An examination of therapist and client behavior in high and low alliance sessions in cognitive-behavioral therapy and process experiential therapy. *Psychotherapy: Theory, Research, Practice and Training, 42*, 297–310.

Westen, D., & Morrison, K. (2001). A multidimensional meta-analysis of treatments for depression, panic, and generalized anxiety disorder: An empirical examination of the status of empirically supported therapies. *Journal of Consulting and Clinical Psychology, 69*(6), 875–899.

Westra, H. A. (2004). Managing resistance in cognitive behavioural therapy: The application of motivational interviewing in mixed anxiety and depression. *Cognitive Behaviour Therapy, 33*, 161–175.

Westra, H. A. (2011). Comparing the predictive capacity of observed in-session resistance to self-reported motivation in cognitive behavioural therapy. *Behavior Research and Therapy, 49*, 106–113.

Westra, H. A., & Arkowitz, H. (2010). Combining motivational interviewing and cognitive-behavioral therapy to increase treatment efficacy for generalized anxiety disorder. In D. Sookman & R. L. Leahy (Eds.), *Treatment resistant anxiety disorders: Resolving impasses to symptom remission* (pp. 199–232). New York: Routledge.

Westra, H. A., Arkowitz, H., & Dozois, D. J. A. (2009). Adding a motivational interviewing pretreatment to cognitive behavioral therapy for generalized anxiety disorder: A preliminary randomized controlled trial. *Journal of Anxiety Disorders, 23*, 1106–1117.

Westra, H. A., Aviram, A., Barnes, M., & Angus, L. (2010). Therapy was not what I expected: A grounded theory analysis of discordance between client expectations and experience of cognitive behavioural therapy. *Psychotherapy Research, 20*, 436–446.

Westra, H. A., Aviram, A. & Doell, F. (2011). Extending motivational interviewing to the treatment of major mental health problems: Current directions and evidence. *Canadian Journal of Psychiatry 56*(11), 643–650.

Westra, H. A., Constantino, M. J., & Aviram, A. (2011). The impact of alliance ruptures on client outcome expectations in cognitive behavioral therapy. *Psychotherapy Research, 21*(4), 472–481.

Westra, H. A., & Dozois, D. J. A. (2006). Preparing clients for cognitive behavioral therapy: A randomized pilot study of motivational interviewing for anxiety. *Cognitive Therapy and Research, 30,* 481–498.

Wilson, G. T., & Schlam, T. R. (2004). The transtheoretical model and motivational interviewing in the treatment of eating and weight disorders. *Clinical Psychology Review, 24,* 361–378.

Zerler, H. (2009). Motivational interviewing in the assessment and management of suicidality. *Journal of Clinical Psychology, 65,* 1207–1217.

Zuroff, D. C., Koestner, R., Moskowitz, D. S., McBride, C., Marshall, M., & Bagby, R. M. (2007). Autonomous motivation for therapy: A new common factor in brief treatments for depression. *Psychotherapy Research, 17*(2), 137–147.

Index